BUT WHAT DOES SCIENCE SAY?

Dr Manan Vora is a double board-certified orthopaedic surgeon, sports medicine specialist, and health and longevity educator, as well as the co-founder of the nutrition company NutriByte Wellness. Additionally, he is also a strategic partner and adviser to various health-tech start-ups because why have just one career when you can have five? If that wasn't enough, he has also collected diplomas and fellowships from around the globe like they are Pokémon cards, and also won the prestigious Edinburgh Surgery Global Scholar Award from the Royal College of Surgeons, Edinburgh, along the way.

When he is not treating joint pains and soothing sore muscles, Dr Vora is busy being a health influencer with a social media following of over half a million! His Instagram, LinkedIn and YouTube are treasure troves of fitness tips, joint health advice and longevity mantras with a sprinkling of humour— because who said doctors can't be funny? Dr Vora is known for saying, 'Your age is a lie!' which makes people rethink their life choices, and well, their gym memberships.

A TEDx and Josh Talks speaker, Dr Vora has won multiple health influencer awards, including the Health Influencer of the Year by the Integrated Health and Wellbeing Council, supported by NITI Aayog and the National Health Authority, Government of India. Dr Vora has spoken at numerous medical conferences as well as corporate events, sharing his expertise on everything from orthopaedic and sports injuries to workplace wellness.

His day is incomplete without dedicating ninety minutes to his workout at the gym and another ninety minutes to spending time with his loved ones at home. If you're looking for a dose of health advice with a side of wit, Dr Vora is your go-to expert. Just don't ask him how he finds the time to do it all—he's too busy living his best life and helping you live yours. *But What Does Science Say?* is his first book.

ADVANCE PRAISE FOR THE BOOK

'In today's world, it's easy to get overwhelmed by all the health advice out there. This book is a breath of fresh air'—**Dr Pal Manickam, gastroenterologist and holistic health content creator**

'[An] absolute must-read for every Indian! This book is an eye-opener, and I learnt so much from it. It's a game changer for anyone who wants to separate health fact from fiction. With clear explanations and scientific literature, it dismantles myths that have misled us for years. An essential guide for better health decisions. I highly recommend people from all age groups to read this book!'—**Revant Himatsingka (Food Pharmer), health content creator and author**

'You got to love Dr Vora's science-based content backed by fun jokes, answering some of the most common health questions we ask on Google!'—**Dr Tanaya Narendra (Dr Cuterus), embryologist, sexual health content creator and author**

'In an age where health misinformation spreads faster than ever, this book serves as a vital corrective. As a doctor, I value the clear, science-based explanations that debunk myths and clarify truths that are critical to good health. It's a must-read for anyone serious about cutting through the noise and understanding what truly matters when it comes to their health and well-being'—**Dr Santhosh Jacob, orthopaedic surgeon and health content creator**

'A must-read. In the world of WhatsApp university and fakefluencers, Dr Manan uses science to bring truth to the surface, something very few do. Get ready to have your myths debunked'—**Prashant Desai, health content creator**

'As a paediatrician, I know how important it is for parents to make the best choices for their child's health, but misinformation can make that difficult. This book busts myths that could affect your child's well-being, offering clear, science-based facts that every parent should know. It offers clarity and empowers families to make better health decisions for their little ones'—**Dr Arpit Gupta, paediatrician and health content creator**

'I'm a doctor and most of the content I create is around busting common myths that Indians have been led to believe for years now. And there's no stopping. There's still a majority that believes in things they see on the internet. Trust me when I say this—we needed something that collated everything in one place and provided evidence-based information. This book is that one resource for you! You NEED to read it!'—**Dr Siddhant Bhargava, clinical nutritionist, health content creator and author**

'This book is an absolute eye-opener for ages thirteen and above! It's not only packed with brilliant science-backed information, but also has a fun, witty and humorous element. The book helps you learn AND teach; I can vouch for it as a doctor. Read it!'—**Dr Divya Vora, gynaecologist and women's health content creator**

BUT WHAT DOES SCIENCE SAY?

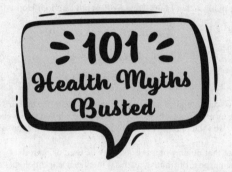

101
Health Myths
Busted

DR MANAN VORA

EBURY
PRESS

An imprint of Penguin Random House

EBURY PRESS

Ebury Press is an imprint of the Penguin Random House group of companies
whose addresses can be found at global.penguinrandomhouse.com

Published by Penguin Random House India Pvt. Ltd
4th Floor, Capital Tower 1, MG Road,
Gurugram 122 002, Haryana, India

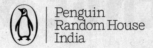

Penguin
Random House
India

First published in Ebury Press by Penguin Random House India 2024

ISBN 9780143466277

Typeset in Bembo Std by Manipal Technologies Limited, Manipal
Printed at Thomson Press India Ltd, New Delhi

www.penguin.co.in

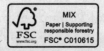

MIX
Paper | Supporting
responsible forestry
FSC® C010615

Dedicated to my mother, Sonal Vora, an exemplary doctor and medical research scientist, whose love and guidance still light my path, even from beyond

Contents

Introduction

We're living in the age of information overload, aren't we? Everywhere you look, there's advice on everything under the sun. But here's the catch: too much information can sometimes leave us more confused than ever!

So, I thought, why not take on the challenge? In this book, I've handpicked 101 health topics, sifted through the noise and analysed the facts. Only to spill the beans on the ultimate truth and introduce you to science—the real superhero of our life.

Science isn't just for lab coats and test tubes. It's in EVERYTHING we do, every single day.

Think about it: From turning milk into yoghurt to making those fluffy bread rolls with yeast. Even our cars, buses, laptops, AirPods and mobile phones . . . yup, all science!

Ever wondered how your GPS gets you everywhere? Science, my friend, science! It's in all things, from counting your steps to tracking your sleep. Even your music streaming is because of science!

Packed with anecdotes and real-life incidents, this book is your ticket to the other side of the story. Here, for every question, science has an answer.

This book is your ultimate guide to separating fact from fiction, truth from myth and science from superstition. It will help you navigate through the maze of health advice out there. It's all about getting to know your body better, understanding exactly what you're putting into it and making informed decisions that pave the way to a healthier life. With a dash of humour and a ton of valuable information, this book will empower you to make smarter choices about your health and well-being.

Whether you're looking to bust common health myths, dive into the world of nutrition or explore the latest fitness trends, consider this book your go-to resource for ALL things health-related. Get ready to take charge of your body and embark on a journey to a happier, healthier you!

As a doctor passionate about debunking health myths, I've covered a wide array of topics in my book. From general health to bone and joint health, I've delved into the importance of maintaining overall well-being. I've also tackled myths surrounding substances like sugar, caffeine and alcohol, shedding light on their effects on the body. Fitness enthusiasts will find valuable insights into workout routines, injury prevention and the truth behind popular exercise myths.

When it comes to nutrition, I've explored the role of various foods and supplements in supporting optimal health, from the benefits of leafy greens to the truth about vitamin supplements. Additionally, I've addressed reproductive health, including common misconceptions about contraception, fertility and sexual health. I've covered women's health and discussed specific topics like menstrual health, pregnancy and menopause. Skin and hair health myths are also debunked, along with valuable tips for maintaining a healthy complexion and luscious locks. Lastly, I've delved into mental health, emphasizing the importance of destigmatizing mental illness and seeking support when needed.

No matter your age or gender, this book has something for everyone! Whether you're a health-conscious teen, a busy parent or a seasoned senior, there's valuable information here that you and your friends can benefit from.

This book is the ultimate gift for kids, teens, friends and family. Whether it's for birthdays, festivals, anniversaries, special occasions or even as return gifts, this treasure trove of knowledge will enrich their lives in ways that last a lifetime. Give the gift of wisdom and insight and watch as it becomes a cherished source of enlightenment and growth for those you care about.

Reading this book isn't just about gaining valuable insights into health and well-being; it's also a surefire way to become the life of the party or a gathering. Armed with the wealth of knowledge and research-backed facts in these pages, you'll be everyone's favourite conversation starter at social gatherings. Whether you're debunking common health myths or sharing fascinating tidbits about nutrition, fitness and general well-being, you'll captivate your audience with your newfound wisdom. Who knew that learning about health could be this much fun?

In the playful adventure of decoding health myths, there's no set path, no rules and certainly no particular way to read this book. You can start wherever you like, with whichever topic is closest to your heart and mind. Flip the pages and read about the myths that intrigue you the most. Leave bookmarks, scribble notes or mark the pages—it's your guide, after all!

Open it to any page and you'll find yourself immersed in a world of health truths, debunking myths left, right and centre. Whether you're a cover-to-cover reader or a random-page opener, this book promises an eye-opening journey into the world of science-backed health facts, wrapped in a blanket of humour and wit.

The next time you come across a WhatsApp forward promising miraculous healing, an Instagram reel making you doubt your food choices or even those so-called well-wishers giving health advice at every turn, grab this book for the real truth.

Let the myth-busting adventure begin!

Crackonomics 101

The Mechanics of Knuckle Popping

Myth: Cracking knuckles can cause arthritis.
'Don't crack your knuckles, your fingers will become weak.'

'It is inauspicious to crack your knuckles.'

If you too have been hearing these admonitions since childhood, let me put your fears to rest once and for all.

But before that, some science. Cracking knuckles is nothing but putting pressure on your fingers or stretching them. It is a activity done unthinkingly, out of habit, boredom, stress or nervousness. It is such a common habit that close to 45 per cent people crack their knuckles.[1] Some people claim to do it to relax the joints; others do it simply for the sound.

The music it creates is definitely satisfying, isn't it?

Well, the reasons people do this are as numerous as the emotions they experience after doing it.

To explain it in medical terms, the human body has 206 bones. Ligaments hold these bones together to create joints. The joints on our hands are called synovial joints and are surrounded by the synovial fluid for lubrication. This fluid is made up of gases, among which nitrogen is in the highest quantity. These gases create bubbles in our joints.

When you put pressure on your fingers, or stretch them, a negative pressure is created, causing a cavity in those joints.[2]

You guessed it—the pop you hear each time you crack your knuckles is the sound of gas bubbles bursting due to pressure.

So why does cracking your knuckles feel so good? Because the joints have been stretched (as an aside, stretching is always a good thing to do, irrespective of the body part).

In simple terms, cracking knuckles does not cause arthritis.[3]

Turns out, all those knuckle cracks weren't breaking your fingers—they were just breaking old myths!

The Multivitamin Mirage

Debunking Daily Dose Dogma

Three of my colleagues and I were heading to Delhi for an important seminar. While waiting at the airport for boarding to commence, I ran into a family friend, Deepak Kumar, who seemed flustered. When I inquired, he mentioned he had forgotten to bring his medications. Reacting quickly, I suggested he retrieve the prescription on his phone so he could purchase them upon reaching the other city he was travelling to.

However, he responded, 'I take them without prescriptions. They're multivitamins, essential for someone of my age!'

It was a classic facepalm moment for me. To give you some context, Deepak is in his late thirties. I can't help but be amazed when well-educated, well-travelled folks like him fall for these internet gimmicks. I swiftly checked his flight details and breathed a sigh of relief when I realized we were on the same plane. It seemed like Deepak was in for a crash course in science today.

Did You Know?

An increasing number of individuals in good health are turning to dietary supplements. However, there is scant evidence to suggest that they guard against diseases.[1]

Supplements help fix micronutrient deficiency or in simpler terms, they ensure you get enough nutrients. But most over-the-counter supplements are taken by people who don't have any obvious signs of lacking nutrients. While there is no proof that these supplements help prevent[2] diseases in healthy people, they do help seniors[3] improve their memory.

Moreover, there's no scientific evidence that consuming certain nutrients[4] is good for health.

As our boarding call echoed through the airport, I walked along with Deepak to the plane. I planned to exchange my seat with the person who would be sitting next to him as I had a burning desire to enlighten him about the fallacies of multivitamins and their empty assurances.

Sometimes, it's so exasperating that I feel like grabbing the other person by the shoulders, shaking them and shouting, 'THIS IS NOT TRUE!'

Upon reaching the tarmac, we observed our plane undergoing refuelling. It dawned on me at that moment. With a firm grip on Deepak's hand, I presented the scene to him as we ascended the stairs. While awaiting entry, I whispered into his ears, 'Just like a plane is refuelled only when it needs to, we should take vitamins only when they are truly needed.'

He stared at me wide-eyed and said, 'Vitamins are safe, Manan. They cannot cause any harm.'

'No, Deepak. Any dose of vitamins A, E, D, C and folic acid without proper advice from a doctor is not advisable because they can potentially harm one's health.[5] And in any case, they may not always be effective in preventing diseases.'

Vitamin supplementation is recommended in conditions where a deficiency is present due to limited access to certain foods, imbalanced diets or poor absorption.[6]

Soon, we reached his seat. Before leaving, I said, 'And if you're really concerned about those vitamins, why don't you see me once you're back? We'll schedule a full body check-up for you and get the proper diagnosis. It's the safest way to get your daily dose of vitamins.[7]

As soon as he settled into his seat, he pulled out his phone. I immediately interrupted him, saying, 'Deepak, don't worry. Our moms are together at a gathering. They know we're on this flight together.'

His reply brought a smile to my face. 'Oh, I was just about to call my wife. She must be arranging my medications for Delhi as I had asked. Let me tell her not to bother anymore.'

At that moment, another passenger approached, indicating that the seat next to Deepak belonged to him. I stepped aside as Deepak appeared to have grasped the lesson well. He didn't seem to require any further tutorials.

Sunscreen

Not Just for Sunny Days, but for Every Shade of Cloud

Last-minute work obligations forced me to cancel our planned couples' trip to the Maldives with two of my friends and their spouses. However, upon their return, we reunited at one of their homes, eager to catch up. Laughter filled the air and our excitement to see each other again was palpable.

As I sat across from my friends, I couldn't help but ask the predictable question: 'How was the Maldives?'

Aman's laughter boomed before he responded, 'Oh, it was amazing, Manan. But let me tell you, we probably spent more on my wife Ritika's sunscreen than the entire trip itself!'

'No way! Don't exaggerate. I am sure the food bill was way higher, with all the exotic delicacies you wanted to keep trying,' Ritika argued as the others laughed.

Aman immediately countered, 'I am not exaggerating at all!'

And then he looked at us and said, 'You have no idea. My wife is absolutely obsessed with sunscreens. I mean, even on cloudy days, she was slathering it on and reapplying it throughout the day like her life depended on it.' He nodded, still chuckling.

'Every few hours, she would be like . . .' He proceeded to mimic her, pretending to take the sunscreen from her bag and apply it over the exposed parts of her body while the rest of us giggled along with Ritika.

'Well, you know, she's not wrong. Sunscreen is crucial for skin protection, especially in places like the Maldives, where the sun can be quite intense,' I said as soon as the laughter subsided.

All eyes were on me as Aman was taken aback. 'Oh? Is it really that important? I always thought it was just to prevent sunburn.'

'You might be surprised to learn how important it is!' I smiled.

Sunscreen helps protect your skin from harmful UV rays, which can cause sunburn, premature ageing and even skin cancer. It's like armour for your skin, shielding it from the sun's damaging effects.[1]

Contrary to reports, sunscreen application has no harmful effects[2] on the skin or on overall health.

Applying sunscreen again[3] ensures that its protective layer remains effective. Rain or shine, indoors or outdoors, sunscreen is the VIP guest on every occasion. Whether you're sipping chai in your pyjamas or conquering the great outdoors, sunscreen is your trusty sidekick![4]

With every passing statement, I could see Ritika's smile getting wider and wider till she finally told him, 'See, I told you!'

He laughed, shaking his head in amusement. 'Well, I guess I'll never understand your fascination with sunscreen, but I'll definitely appreciate it more now.'

I added, 'If you ask me, I am glad to know that she is taking her skin health seriously, even if it means spending a small fortune on sunscreen. After all, when it comes to protecting your skin, a little extra investment is always worth it in the long run.'

Ritika, who was in her element now, said, 'Unlike some investments that can sink faster than the *Titanic*, investing in sunscreen is like having a life raft for your skin. It'll keep you afloat through sunny days and stormy weather!' And then she winked at Aman, whose poor investment decisions were legendary.

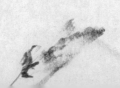

Gym Fears and Family Tears

A Comedy of Cardio Catastrophes

As a seasoned member of our family WhatsApp group, I had grown accustomed to the occasional influx of forwarded messages, ranging from earnest warnings about the latest online scams to heartwarming tales of stray puppies finding forever homes. However, nothing could have prepared me for the bombshell that landed in our virtual midst one fine morning.

Amid the usual flurry of good morning wishes and emoji-laden banter, a distant relative—let's call him Uncle Gyanesh—dropped a link to a study claiming that hitting the gym could lead to heart disease. Cue the panic-inducing chain of comments as Uncle Gyanesh proceeded to tag every gym-goer and fitness enthusiast in our family tree, urging them to steer clear of those treacherous treadmills and weight machines.

Now, as the self-appointed guardian of sanity and science in our digital family hub, I couldn't let this slide without a healthy dose of sarcasm and a sprinkle of sass.

'Oh my gosh!' I began, my fingers itching to lob some truth bombs into the sea of alarmist emojis. 'So apparently, hitting the gym is now akin to volunteering for a heart attack. Who knew those innocent dumbbells and elliptical machines were secretly plotting our demise?'

As I proceeded to dismantle Uncle Gyanesh's dubious claims with a flurry of facts and logic, I couldn't help but inject a healthy dose of sarcasm into my rebuttal.

Gymming does not lead to a heart attack. On the contrary, it can save you from one.[1]

Did You Know?

Lack of physical activity, along with high blood pressure, abnormal blood lipid levels, smoking and obesity, is among the top five major risk factors for cardiovascular disease.[2]

Regular exercise can counter the risk factors for cardiovascular disease. For instance, it helps with weight loss and can lower blood pressure. Exercise also lowers 'bad' cholesterol and total cholesterol while increasing 'good' cholesterol. In diabetic individuals, exercise improves the body's ability to use insulin to control blood sugar levels. Although the impact of exercise may seem small, when combined with other lifestyle changes like healthy eating, quitting smoking and medication, consistent, moderate exercise can significantly reduce overall cardiovascular risk.[3]

In short, exercise isn't just a workout—it's a cardio party for your heart, complete with confetti and disco lights.[4]

With each witty retort and sarcastic quip, I watched as the tension in the chat gradually dissolved into laughter and light-hearted banter. Even Uncle Gyanesh, bless his sceptical soul, couldn't help but chuckle at the absurdity of his own doing.

Here are five tips to stay safe while working out:

1. **Regular check-ups:** If you are over fifty or have a strenuous routine, consult a cardiologist for regular tests.
2. **Listen to your body:** Avoid overdoing exercise; quality over quantity is key.
3. **Timing matters:** Don't exercise immediately after eating.
4. **Stay hydrated:** Keep yourself hydrated before, during and after workouts.
5. **No steroids:** Say no to steroids; they are not worth the risk.

Pushing yourself too hard during workouts can leave you in oxygen debt, causing your heart to throw a tantrum like a malfunctioning disco ball. To dodge this disco disaster, just be a little more mindful. Sure, scary incidents can happen, but throwing in the sweat towel isn't the solution!

As I signed off with a flourish, suggesting a group workout session complete with synchronized sofa squats and remote-control curls, I thought about the absurdity of it all. In a world filled with internet rumours and fitness fads,

sometimes the best defence is a healthy dose of humour—
and a willingness to laugh in the face of fear.

And who knows, maybe one day Uncle Gyanesh will
trade in his scepticism for a pair of gym shorts and join us
for a round of cardio comedy. Until then, we'll just keep
sweating out the silliness, one hilarious WhatsApp exchange
at a time.

Feast or Famine

Debunking Intermittent Fasting Myths

n the middle of a typical day at work, I encountered Almas, a twenty-nine-year-old grappling with Type 2 diabetes and struggling with weight issues. During our consultation, Almas candidly shared her myriad challenges with me. I suggested that she explore intermittent fasting (IF) as a potential weight loss strategy, along with a few other lifestyle modifications. Additionally, I recommended a session with a nutritionist to help her identify suitable dietary choices to support her fitness goals.

Despite her upbeat demeanour throughout our conversation, I noticed a shift in Almas's expression when I broached the topic of IF. Sensing her apprehension, I inquired, 'Is there a problem, Almas? We can always tailor our approach to accommodate your habits and lifestyle. Please feel free to share your concerns.'

Almas hesitated before responding, 'Well, Doctor, I've heard some scary stories about intermittent fasting. People say it's quite extreme and can be harmful. I'm not sure if it's the right approach for me.'

13

I nodded understandingly. 'I appreciate your honesty, Almas. It's important to consider all perspectives before making any decisions. However, it's worth noting that intermittent fasting can be approached in various ways, and we can customize a plan that suits your needs and comfort level.'

Almas still seemed sceptical. 'Recently, I read that intermittent fasting is bad for the heart too. Actually, nothing that I have heard about it is good. Low energy levels. Constant fatigue!'

'No, Almas,' I reassured her. 'Intermittent fasting is a great way to lose weight.[1] And no, it does not impact your heart badly. On the contrary, it lowers the risk of cardiovascular diseases.[2]

Contrary to popular belief, intermittent fasting is not a starvation diet. It's a pattern of eating that involves alternating periods of eating and fasting, which can have numerous health benefits.[3] It works by restricting the timing of food intake, which helps create a calorie deficit and may enhance metabolic flexibility, leading to potential weight loss and other health benefits.

IF is highly effective when it comes to losing fat mass.[4] It also results in reduced overall calorie consumption, enhanced insulin sensitivity and alterations in several hormones responsible for controlling appetite and energy equilibrium.[5]

'But won't skipping meals slow the metabolism and leave me feeling weak?' Almas was not convinced.

I shook my head. 'Intermittent fasting can boost your metabolism and promote fat burning.[6] And as for feeling weak, it's all about timing your meals and ensuring you get enough nutrients during your eating window.'

Contrary to popular belief, people experience increased energy and mental clarity[7] during fasting periods. IF is the best way to give your body a break from constant digestion and allow it to tap into its fat stores for fuel. It promotes gut health[8] by allowing the digestive system time to rest and repair. It also supports liver function[9] by reducing fat accumulation and promoting detoxification.

While IF is commonly used for weight loss, research also indicates its benefits in enhancing brain function, promoting self-healing through autophagy, lowering blood sugar, decreasing inflammation and enhancing metabolic adaptability.[10]

I asked Almas, 'What do you think about scheduling a follow-up meeting in two weeks instead of four? This way, if you encounter any challenges with intermittent fasting, we can address them promptly.'

Finally, she smiled. 'Yes, that sounds doable. I can try it for a few days and see how my body responds, rather than completely writing it off based on hearsay.'

After a brief pause, Almas continued, 'Thank you so much, Doctor! This discussion has put my fears to rest. I am no longer apprehensive about trying IF to lose weight.'

The smile on her face was a huge relief to me as it gave me hope that science would always be the light at the end of the dark tunnel of myths and misinformation.

Hot and Cold Confusion

Unravelling the Ankletastrophe

As the beats of the *dhol* reverberated through the air and the scent of marigolds mingled with laughter, I found myself swept up in the whirlwind of my friend Sajid's wedding celebrations. But being a doctor, I couldn't help but be on call even during festivities.

It was during the *sangeet* night that the unexpected happened. Amid the frenzied dancing, one of our dear friends, Rahul, missed a step and tumbled to the ground with a yelp of pain. As we gathered around him, concern etched on our faces, someone suggested, 'Quick, get a hot water bag to ease the pain!'

I couldn't help but chuckle inwardly as I stepped forward. 'Hold on, hold on,' I said, 'Let me handle this. Can someone please get an ice pack for Rahul?'

'Why an ice pack? What he needs is a hot water bag right now . . .' a voice suggested from the crowd, which I deliberately ignored.

After a bit of coaxing, we managed to get Rahul seated comfortably. I then proceeded to enlighten my friends about the age-old debate of ice versus heat for injuries.

'You see,' I began, 'if you twist your ankle or injure yourself in any way, the immediate go-to isn't a heating pad, but ice.'

Blank looks greeted me along with a chorus of protests. 'But Doc, heat is supposed to soothe the pain, right?'

I nodded, a mischievous glint in my eye. 'Ah, but in this case, ice is your best friend. It helps to reduce swelling and numbs the area, providing immediate relief[1]

By that time, the cold pack had arrived. As we applied ice to his ankle, Rahul let out a sigh of relief, the pain visibly subsiding.

While using cold therapy usually helps reduce swelling a bit, it doesn't speed up recovery. Ice does help restrict swelling, especially in cases where too much swelling can hinder the healing process, as in severe joint sprains.[2]

'I'm so confused about when to use ice and when to use heat for an injury,' someone from the group rued.

I clarified, 'Yeah, it can be tricky. But here's the deal: for acute injuries, like if you suddenly twist your ankle, always go for ice. It helps constrict blood vessels, numb the pain and reduce swelling.'

'Got it. What about chronic injuries, like muscle sprains and joint aches?' a senior member asked.

'For those, you want to go with heat, like a hot water bottle. It boosts blood circulation and eases muscle spasms, making the pain more manageable,' I explained.

Amid nods of understanding, I couldn't resist injecting a bit of laughter into the situation. 'But remember, folks, we're not trying to cook a biryani here! Moderation is key when applying heat.'

With Rahul now on the road to recovery and the mood lightened by my impromptu medical lecture, we resumed our revelry with even more gusto. The dhol beats seemed to throb with renewed energy and laughter filled the air once more.

Black Hair Today, Gone Tomorrow

The Truth of Grey Hair Multiplication

I t was one of those raucous family gatherings where every corner echoed with laughter and chatter. Exuberantly catching up with relatives, I spotted my cousin Riya looking somewhat downcast in the jubilant crowd. As I approached her, I couldn't help but notice her hair, which seemed to have acquired a light shade of grey, premature for someone in her early twenties.

'Hey, Riya, what's up? Why the long face?' I asked.

She sighed, running her fingers through her silver-streaked locks. 'Oh, Manan *bhai*, it's my hair. It's turned grey and the grey is spreading like wildfire! I don't know what to do.'

Riya went on to tell me how she had spotted one grey hair a couple of months ago and decided to pluck it. Since then, the number of her grey hair had just been multiplying.

I decided to delve deeper into the mystery of her prematurely greying hair. 'Hold on a sec, Riya. Let me get this straight. You're telling me that you think plucking one grey hair has sparked a full-blown rebellion of silver strands on your head?'

She nodded solemnly, looking utterly perplexed. 'Yes, it's like they're multiplying overnight! I don't understand what's happening.'

Our conversation was already earning a few curious glances from nearby relatives. I took her aside and said, 'Oh, Riya, you sweet summer child! That is not how our hair works.'

Taking a deep breath to compose myself, I launched into a mock tirade against the absurd notion that plucking one grey hair leads to its proliferation.

'Listen, Riya, believe me when I say that grey hair isn't contagious. It's not like a Bollywood dance number in which one dancer infects the rest with their moves! Medically, it's impossible to pluck a single grey hair and trigger the growth of more grey hairs from the same follicle. Each follicle typically produces only one hair. Plucking one grey hair won't induce the surrounding hair to turn grey; greying is linked primarily to melanin changes within each individual hair.[1]

Riya's eyes widened in surprise and she let out a nervous giggle at my analogy. 'But then why is this happening to me, Manan bhai? Is there something wrong with me?'

I placed a comforting hand on her shoulder, adopting a mock-serious expression. 'Why *fikar*, when Manan is here?' And then I explained the mystery of the premature greying of hair.

There are multiple reasons for this phenomenon, like stress, genetics, nutritional deficiencies . . . the list goes on.

In most cases, genetics may be the predominant factor behind the premature greying of hair. Research has also indicated the involvement of smoking and deficiencies.[2] Even autoimmune conditions[3] like vitiligo, pernicious anaemia, autoimmune thyroid disorders and Werner's syndrome lead to premature greying of hair. Some studies have also suggested that environmental factors[4] like ultraviolet light exposure and climate, medication use and inadequate nutrition also contribute to premature greying of hair.

Her face brightened slightly as she absorbed my words. 'So you mean to tell me that I'm not doomed to resemble a distinguished elder statesman before my time?'

'Exactly!' I said. 'But remember, rather than resorting to remedies based on superstition, it's best to consult a good dermatologist who can diagnose the root cause of your greying hair and prescribe a suitable treatment.'

Just then, the sound of a popular Bollywood track blared from the speakers, prompting nearby relatives to start dancing vigorously. 'Hey, Riya, let's forget about your hair woes for now and join in the fun! Who knows, maybe a few dance moves will chase away those grey hairs!' I suggested with a grin.

Riya laughed, the tension dissipating from her features. 'You're right, Manan bhai. Let's show them how it's done!'

And with that, we threw caution to the wind and joined the impromptu dance party, leaving Riya's grey hair conundrum to be solved another day—preferably by a qualified dermatologist and not by plucking each silver strand in sight!

Organic

Nature's Overrated Label

A new couple had recently moved in next door. My wife bumped into our new neighbours a couple of times and got invited for a cup of tea—with me, of course! So one Saturday afternoon, we found ourselves sitting in their living room exchanging pleasantries.

Before long, our neighbours appeared with trays adorned with snacks, complemented by freshly brewed coffee. While I adhered to my usual cup of hot java, the others indulged in cold coffee to combat the heat. As I glanced at the array of snacks, I couldn't help but exchange a knowing look with my wife.

Our neighbour, whom we'll refer to as T, noticed my discomfort and reassured me, saying, 'Oh, don't worry! They're all organic. I recall your wife mentioning your healthy eating habits.' Her husband joined in, emphasizing how they, too, were very mindful of their dietary choices and bought only organic food items.

I couldn't contain myself any longer; I just had to vent. I took a sip of my black coffee to muster up some internal courage and blurted out, 'I hate to be the bearer of bad news, but . . . the belief that organic food is inherently healthier is just a myth.[1]

My wife, who was accustomed to such discussions with me, took her cold coffee and settled comfortably on the couch, ready to enjoy the show. Her expression practically screamed, 'Let the show begin!'

So I started doing what I enjoy most—debunking myths and shedding light on the science behind health.

I quickly gulped my espresso and said, 'From a medical standpoint, there's no concrete evidence of organic food having any significant impact on health.[2] However, mentally, it's a fantastic stimulant! It convinces you that you've made a supremely healthy food choice.[3] But beyond that placebo effect, nada!'

In a study, it was also found that transitioning to organic foods coincided with other healthy lifestyle adjustments. Hence, attributing the observed effects solely to organic food was not entirely conclusive.[4] Consumers opt for organic food under the belief that it is naturally produced, safe, healthy and of superior quality.[5]

People often choose organic food due to the considerations of human health, food safety, attitudes, perceptions and a willingness to pay a premiuim.[6] However, even the promise of food safety is dubious, despite these products having a premium charge. Recent cases of contaminated organic food have brought to light concerns about the safety and risks associated with organic produce.[7]

'You know the saying, "Never judge a book by its cover"? Well, the same goes for food. Just because something is labelled "organic" doesn't mean it's automatically top-notch quality.' I uttered those words to the sound of a crunch and looked up to find T paused midway through a bite of the organic cookies, processing the new information.

She left the cookie half-eaten, looking somewhat sheepish. 'One cookie won't make a difference, T. Go ahead and finish it,' I said with a grin.

T's husband, looking puzzled, chimed in, 'I'm so confused about what's right and what's not. Grocery shopping has become so stressful, bro!'

'Just think of the grocery items as Poo from *Kabhi Khushi Kabhie Gham*,' I said and did my best Kareena Kapoor imitation to say, '*Kaun hai yeh jisne dobara mudke mujhe nahi dekha?* (who is this who hasn't turned around to look at me again)?'

The blank look on each one's face confirmed that my joke hadn't landed. So I rephrased it. 'Pick up any grocery item and turn it around to read the ingredients listed. That is the best way to determine if they are actually organic or not.'

Right on cue, T and her husband burst into laughter, amused by my belated attempt at humour.

Burning Fat

Hitting the Bull's Eye with Weight Loss

One weekend, we all gathered at my childhood friend Adil's house to celebrate the exciting news of his finalized wedding dates. While sipping glasses of home-made aam panna to beat the heat, we playfully teased Adil while also discussing plans for the wedding festivities three months later.

Among discussions of an all-boys road trip to Goa and shopping, Nasser suddenly stood up and exclaimed, 'Bro, I think you should do something about that double chin! Your close-ups will be ruined by that weak jawline.'

Adil, who had been calmly sipping his aam panna until then, suddenly turned to face the mirror behind him, cupped his face with both hands and adopted a serious expression. 'You're absolutely right, bro! Imagine the number of pictures and videos zooming into my tiniest expressions—with this! I need to get rid of this.'

Rehaan suggested, 'I know someone who teaches face sculpting exercises to get that perfect jawline. I can connect you with them!'

Adil was excited. 'Oh yes, please do that.'

Many of us nodded in agreement as he scanned the room and asked, 'What do you guys think?'

When his gaze landed on me, I knew it was my turn to speak.

'Bhai Adil, I'm all for getting fit. But sorry to burst your bubble, you can't just target your fat burn like that.'

'But . . . I have seen those face sculpting exercises show results, with people getting chiselled jawlines in a few months,' Rehaan's hesitation conveyed his confusion clearly.

'You're not alone, bro . . . It's a common myth and has no scientific backing.[1] Spot reduction[2] also humorously termed "magic targeting", is a favourite concept because it tickles our fancy. I mean, it makes sense, right? If you're exercising a specific muscle, it should drain the fat around it.'

A study analysed participants for a specific period. MRI scans conducted before and after the programme showed that fat loss was spread out across the body, rather than just around the trained part.[3] And there is a good reason for this.

The fat stored in fat cells is in the form of triglycerides. Muscle cells can't directly use triglycerides for energy—it's like trying to run a car on crude oil. First, the fat needs to be broken down into glycerol and free fatty acids, which then enter the bloodstream. So, during long periods of exercise, the fat used for fuel can come from anywhere in your body, not just the area you're working out.[4]

'Bhai Adil, at the end of the day, it's simple maths— the calories you burn versus the calories you devour, not the number of reps you do at the gym. And trust me, no amount of targeted jumping jacks will outsmart that bag of chips you snuck in last night!' I explained, putting a hand on his shoulder. It took him a moment to catch on, and then he shot me an angry glare.

'*Yaar*, don't reveal all my secrets like this to my wife in the future!'

'Now you are giving us ideas, bro!' Nasser chipped in, making Adil turn red as he chased him around the room.

Rise and Grind

The Breakfast Breakdown

I thoroughly enjoy delving into the history of cities through heritage walks. The stories behind each city never fail to captivate me. Uncovering hidden gems and lesser-known spots always leaves me feeling deeply connected to the city I'm exploring. When I learnt of a heritage walk in Mazgaon showcasing its Chinese village, I knew I couldn't miss it.

I encountered numerous individuals who shared my interests and our time together was enjoyable as we traversed the lanes and streets for nearly an hour and a half, uncovering the hidden stories they held. Everything was going smoothly till we paused for a food break. Sampling local cuisine was an integral part of the walk, and our guide suggested various options for us to try. We split into smaller groups to explore whatever appealed to our tastes.

Shortly afterwards, our conversation turned to the topic of breakfast as we sat down to eat. Aditya, one of the group, expressed his disdain for breakfast, claiming that it made him feel lethargic for the rest of the day. Another member, Shreyas, said he preferred lighter breakfast options such as cereals, poha and upma, eschewing heavier fare like idli, dosa and parathas.

Srishti, also a part of the group, began discussing her breakfast routine. 'I have grown up hearing the age-old adage, "Eat breakfast like a king, lunch like a prince and dinner like a pauper." And I follow this like a faithful Indian child. Even though I have been living on my own for the past five years and it's a struggle most days, I am not ready to let go of it just yet.'

As I ate, I sensed their expectant gazes fixed on me, as though they were waiting for me to contribute to the conversation.

I cleared my throat and began, 'I firmly believe that how one chooses to have breakfast, whether like royalty or like a pauper, is entirely up to the individual's taste buds.' Detecting a shift in the group's atmosphere, I immediately added, 'Don't get me wrong! Breakfast is indeed important. I am not debating that. What I am saying is that having breakfast like a king is not important.'

Whenever someone mentions, 'Eat breakfast like a king,' just ask them, 'Who said that?' You'll quickly realize that science isn't backing up these jokes![1]

The size and composition[2] of breakfast matters more than its extravagance. Contrary to popular belief, a heavy breakfast laden with ghee-soaked parathas or sugary treats may not be the healthiest choice.

A balanced breakfast, comprising whole grains, protein-rich foods like eggs or lentils and plenty of fruits and vegetables, provides sustained energy levels[3] throughout the day. Instead of parathas and pohas, you can explore healthier alternatives such as oatmeal with nuts and seeds, vegetable omelettes or smoothie bowls bursting with fresh flavours.

Moreover, opting for smaller portions helps prevent sluggishness[4] and promotes better digestion. After a lighter, nutrient-dense[5] breakfast, you will feel more energized and focused throughout the day.

'You have got me confused, bro! Should we or should we not have breakfast?' Aditya asked.

'Just be mindful of what you eat. You will notice a positive shift in not only your emotional and physical well-being, but also your stamina. These small changes can make a huge difference to your health as you say hello to an active day and bid goodbye to post-meal lethargy and bloating!'

Shreyas and Srishti spoke at the same time with their mouths stuffed with food, 'So we can eat this puri-bhaji guilt-free!' It sounded gibberish yet made sense. We couldn't help but laugh together.

Puff Fiction

Exposing the Truth About Vaping

While window shopping with my wife one day, I ran into a friend who was shopping for his teenage nephew.

Out of curiosity, I inquired about the gift he had in mind.

'Oh, he's made my job easier. He's asking for a green apple-flavoured vape.'

I responded in disbelief and frustration, 'You can't possibly consider gifting him a vape! It's not a healthy choice.'

'Why? Isn't it a harmless thing?'

'No! Not at all,' I snapped.

His befuddled face was my sign to continue and explain how smoking electronic cigarettes (e-cigs), commonly referred to as 'vaping', is marketed as a safe or less harmful substitute for smoking or as a tool to help quit smoking.[1] Vapes contain inhalants such as nicotine, tetrahydrocannabinol and cannabidiol.[2] These harmful ingredients in e-cigs can be harmful to one's health and even cause death.[3] Regular vaping is also associated with lung disorders in teens and young adults.[4]

'Well, surprise, surprise!' I said to my friend, 'Turns out, it's not just a fun ride for smokers; it's got a VIP pass to addiction[5] and it's dragging the non-smokers[6] into the party too!'

And just to put the cherry on top of my argument, I threw in a little extra at the end by adding that the biggest concern in this area is insufficient research and the absence of clear rules for making e-cigarettes and their vaping liquid.[7]

The expression on his face was one of utter shock. 'Oh my! He's been vaping for a while now, and none of us intervened because we thought it was harmless.'

'Don't beat yourself up. It's all part of the vape companies' masterful plan. They want us to buy into the notion that e-cigarettes are harmless, just because they contain nicotine and not tobacco. Vapes are combustion-free, which is often thought to reduce harmful effects compared to tobacco. However, when scientists tested this claim, they found no scientific evidence to support it. No science is backing that tale up!'[8]

'Recent studies have also shown that the flavourings in e-cigarettes can harm cells.[9] Vaping poses risks which warrant further investigation to develop clear public policy guidance and regulation.'[10]

'Whew! You're my hero, Doc! Imagine the guilt trip I'd be on if I'd gifted him that vape. Dodged a bullet there, but looks like I've just traded one problem for another, huh? Classic me!'

'Can't decide on a gift? No worries! Let's make a trip to the bookstore. You might discover some enlightening reads that debunk all those health myths swirling in your mind!'

Unearthing the Truth

Shilajit's Sperm-Boosting Saga

As I navigated the crowded roads of Mumbai, my friend Rajesh and I found ourselves at a standstill in an unending traffic jam. With nothing to do but wait, our attention was drawn to a towering billboard ahead, its bright colours and bold letters advertising shilajit.

'Wow!' I exclaimed, somewhat irritated, as I took in the imposing advertisement. 'Imagine the money being spent on something like this!'

Rajesh nodded in agreement, his tone tinged with amusement. 'Oh yes, who would have thought a decade ago that this was possible? We are now openly talking about shilajit and products that help male sexual health.'

'That's not what I meant,' I clarified, shaking my head. 'The money spent on a misleading product like this is huge.'

Rajesh's expression shifted to one of curiosity. 'What are you saying?' he asked, prompting me to explain further.

Shilajit is an organic–mineral product of predominantly biological origin, formed in the mountains. Traditionally, it has been considered to be helpful in the prevention of several diseases.[1]

However, it needs to be added that only a purified version of shilajit is suitable for human consumption.[2] Recent research suggests that certain shilajit-based products promoted online contain measurable levels of heavy metals[3] like lead, mercury and arsenic. This may pose risks of intoxication[4] due to the presence of mycotoxins, heavy metal ions, polymeric quinones (oxidant agents) and free radicals, among other substances.

Consuming shilajit without the knowledge of permissible levels of metals is unsafe and could potentially result in serious health issues.[5]

'And I thought it is natural, so it cannot be harmful!' Rajesh confessed.

'I don't blame you, bro! These smartly worded advertisements exploit people's trust in natural medicines by not disclosing all their ingredients, which can result in adverse effects.'[6]

'In a world saturated with information from messaging apps and social media, how do you discern what's beneficial for you and what's harmful?' he sighed.

'It's very simple, if you ask me—WhatsApp forwards and advertisements shouldn't be trusted, especially when it comes to your health and that of your loved ones. If there's a concern, seek advice from a doctor. There are qualified specialists for every medical issue who can provide you with the right treatment. Self-medication can be extremely harmful,' I clarified.

'And it is green!' Rajesh motioned at the green light, which signalled both our movement forward and the resolution of his confusion.

Antibiotics

Anti-heroes or Superheroes?

Each year, just after Diwali, my whole family gets together for a special lunch to celebrate the Hindu New Year. This includes close and extended family members from both sides of the family.

It's a tradition we cherish, a time to come together, wearing crisp, colourful new clothes and sparkling jewellery. The air is filled with joy and excitement as we head to a restaurant where we've booked a huge table just for us. The idea is simple—we want everyone to have a fantastic time without worrying about anything else.

We were all seated around a big table, menus spread out, and everyone was busy deciding what to order. Soon, a waiter placed a plate of crisp fried starters in the centre of the table.

One of my relatives, let's call him Ravi, shook his head, pushed the plate aside and said, 'No, thanks. I'm on antibiotics, so I should avoid fried stuff.'

I couldn't help but raise an eyebrow at his statement. 'What happened? Are you alright?' I asked, a little worried.

For those who might not know, antibiotic treatment is a cornerstone of modern medicine, widely used to combat infections. The success of modern medicine, including organ transplantation, cancer therapy, the management of preterm babies and advanced surgeries, owes much to effective antibiotic treatment, which controls bacterial infections.[1]

Coming back to Ravi, I was genuinely concerned because when we had spoken last month, he had been under medication and taking antibiotics for his persistent dry cough.

Ravi gave a dismissive wave in response to my concern and said, 'Oh, it's just for my cough. Nothing major.'

I almost choked on my drink. 'Didn't you take this last month as well?'

Ravi looked puzzled. 'Oh yes, I did. At that time, I had consulted a doctor who had prescribed this. So last week, when the same symptoms showed up, I decided to repeat the course myself without visiting the doctor again. It did help me immensely last time, so what's the harm?'

I couldn't let this one slide. 'Hmm. Well, Ravi, I think you might have got it wrong there. Taking antibiotics without a doctor's guidance can actually be harmful. It can lead to antibiotic resistance in your body.'

Taking pills without a doctor's advice is like playing Russian roulette with your health. And if antibiotics were a superhero, they'd be called Antibioti-can't, wreaking havoc on your body if you use them without a doctor's supervision (read more about popping pills without a prescription and the impact of that on page 231).

The main cause of the rise of antibiotic resistance is the overuse of antibiotics. While antibiotics kill sensitive bacteria, they allow resistant pathogens to survive and multiply through natural selection. However, in the long run, the bacteria may develop resistance against the antibiotic, which might then have no impact on the infection.[2]

The association between antibiotic resistance and an increased risk of longer hospitalizations and mortality is well established.[3]

Ravi's eyes widened. 'What do you mean?'

'See, antibiotics are like soldiers fighting off an enemy army in your body, which, in this case, are the harmful bacteria causing your infection. Now, taking antibiotics for a short while is like a quick, surgical strike. It takes out the bad guys effectively. But if you keep taking them for too long, the bacteria in your body get smart. They figure out how to fight the antibiotics and the next time you get sick, those antibiotics might not work at all!'[4]

Ravi looked visibly concerned. 'Oh, I had no idea. What do you suggest I do?'

I put a hand on his shoulder to reassure him. 'Let's relish this scrumptious spread for now. Tomorrow, we'll run some routine tests to check the infection. After that, we can consider consulting a specialist.'

The Great Immunity Hoax

Exposing the Truth behind Boosters

As physicians, we frequently receive gifts, often from pharmaceutical and health companies. Imagine my surprise when I found a box of 'immunity boosting' snacks from a company waiting for me on my desk last Diwali. Neatly packaged, the box was colourful and inviting, adorned with images of snacks in different shapes and sizes. The company specialized in snacks that apparently had the ability to enhance consumers' immunity.

I scrutinized it suspiciously, rotating it 360 degrees to peruse their claims, when my assistant entered the room. She was taken aback by my expression and inquired, 'Is everything alright, Doctor? You're eyeing it as if it's a ticking bomb. They are just snacks!'

I sighed. 'I wish spotting trouble was as simple as spotting a ticking snack box!'

My assistant gave me a puzzled look as I motioned for her to take a seat and began: 'Time for a crash course in science and immunity boosters.'

The immune system, led by the white blood cells, a.k.a. immune cells, is like your body's defence team.[1] It's made up of cells, chemicals and processes that protect you from germs, viruses and other harmful stuff that can make you sick.[2] These tiny soldiers are already on duty, fighting 24/7 to keep you healthy. A healthy immune system is important for protection from harmful germs and for tolerating harmless ones, as well as for digesting food and recognizing the body's own cells.[3]

'Well, technically speaking, your body's already got its own immunity superheroes. So those so-called immunity boosters,' I pointed to the box of immunity-boosting snacks, 'are like bringing sand to the beach!' And I added, 'What's worse is that none of these so-called immunity boosters have any real medical effect.'[4]

Immunity-boosting food items are like *Bunty and Babli*. They promise the world, swindle your hard-earned cash and vanish into thin air, leaving you with nothing but buyer's remorse.[5] If you read most of the articles on the internet that talk about immunity-boosting food items, they clearly emphasize eating a healthy diet full of fruits and vegetables to boost your immune system.[6]

It's worth noting that many of the immunity boosters mentioned in these articles aren't mentioned in medical guidelines and come from complementary and alternative medicine. This also applies to some nutritional advice that relies on either limited scientific evidence or traditional medicine.[7]

So what should one rely on for their immunity?

To support your immune system, make sure to eat plenty of essential nutrients and beneficial compounds.[8]

'Should I toss out this box?' she asked hesitantly, eyeing the yellow box full of cookies wrapped in a red bow.

'The snacks inside are tasty and perfectly fine to eat,' I replied. 'Just don't expect them to work miracles on boosting immunity. If we enjoy them with that understanding, there's no need to throw them away.'

With a mischievous grin, I cracked open the box and rescued a tiny packet of baked beetroot chips. Offering her a chip, I took a bite and let the deliciousness drive away the immunity-boosting ghosts.

Laughing Off the Blues

Dispelling the 'Mind over Matter' Misconception!

As the sunlight filtered through the curtains of my clinic, I found myself settling into my usual routine, ready to tackle whatever medical mysteries the day would bring, when an unexpected call from an old patient took me by surprise.

As my phone buzzed with an incoming call, I glanced at the screen to see the familiar name of Pankajbhai, a long-time patient and friend. Curiosity piqued, I answered the call and was greeted by his earnest voice.

'Dr Manan, I need your help,' Pankajbhai began, his tone laden with concern. 'You know my son, Rohan—he's been feeling down lately, saying he's depressed. But I know depression is all in the mind. Can you tell him that in person and set him straight? He has his board exams in a few months and this is impacting his studies!'

I paused, taking a moment to gather my thoughts. It wasn't the first time I had encountered such a misconception about depression, but addressing it always required sensitivity and understanding.

'Pankajbhai,' I replied gently, 'depression is not just a state of mind. It's a medical condition, a disease that can affect anyone, regardless of age or background. Depression is the most frequently studied psychiatric disorder in numerous research studies.[1] Research indicates that depressive disorders cause substantial impairment,[2] disability[3] and reduced quality of life[4] for those affected.'

There was a brief silence on the other end of the line, followed by a hesitant response: 'But . . . How can that be? He seems fine physically. It's all in his head, isn't it?'

I could sense Pankajbhai's reluctance to accept the reality of his son's condition, a sentiment all too common in our society, where mental health issues are often stigmatized or dismissed.

Some factors linked to depression in children include school-related stress, family-related stress and a family history of mental illness. Studies have also found that children with a depressive disorder often have more family members affected by mental illnesses than children without such a disorder. Clinical signs may include less interest in play, increased fatigue, low self-esteem, trouble concentrating, frequent physical complaints, behavioural issues like anger or aggression, declining school performance and suicidal tendencies.[5]

'Think of it this way,' I continued, striving to convey the gravity of the situation. 'Just like diabetes or hypertension, depression is a disorder that requires proper medical attention. Ignoring it won't make it go away.'

There was a hint of resignation in Pankajbhai's voice as he finally relented. 'I suppose you're right, Doctor. So what should I do?'

I tried explaining to him, despite knowing the journey ahead would not be easy. 'The first step is to seek help from a qualified psychiatrist. I can recommend someone who specializes in treating depression. And most importantly, be there for Rohan. Offer him your support and understanding as he navigates this challenging time.'

Additionally, engaging in aerobic exercise,[6] resistance training and mind-body exercises can help alleviate depressive symptoms and improve overall mood.

With a heartfelt 'thank you', Pankajbhai bid me farewell, promising to follow my advice. As I hung up, I couldn't help but reflect on the pervasive misconceptions surrounding mental health in our society (read about the other misconceptions about mental health on page 73).

It was a reminder of the importance of education and empathy when it came to addressing such issues. While the road to acceptance and healing might be fraught with obstacles, it was heartening to know that Pankajbhai was willing to take the first step towards helping his son.

As I turned my attention back to my patients, I resolved to continue advocating for mental health awareness, one conversation at a time. After all, healing began not just with medication, but with understanding and compassion.

Unmasking the Invisible Enemy

The Real Scoop on Toilet Seats

My friends Rakhi and Jigar were known for throwing the most unforgettable parties. To celebrate Rakhi's thirtieth birthday, they hosted a themed party where guests were asked to come dressed as their favourite funny characters. For the occasion, I chose to dress up as Rosesh Sarabhai.

Running into old and new friends at the party was a blast. Trying to guess their characters and watching them act them out was the icing on the cake for the evening.

I ran into Fatema, a dear old friend now based in Dubai. We embraced, and I jokingly said, 'Finally, we met! We were supposed to catch up three weeks ago. How's your trip been so far?'

She chuckled and said, 'Look at you! You've picked the perfect character. It suits you to a T!' I retorted, 'Well, *Jab We Met's* Geet does complete justice to you too!'

For a moment, it felt like the good old times in high school, when we studied together. I brought her back to the present with a hard-hitting question, 'So, tell me. How are things? Where have you been? How is India treating you after a decade now?'

'You won't believe it! As soon as I arrived, we had to visit my grandmother. We took a road trip to get there, and during the journey, I had to use one of those roadside restrooms. Ever since then, I've been dealing with a severe UTI. *Dost*, I only started feeling better earlier this week, and I decided to come to this party so I could catch up with everyone. The past few weeks have been tough, recovering from this awful UTI. I didn't even have the energy to reach out to anyone.'

'Oh no, that sounds terrible! I can't imagine how uncomfortable that must have been. But I'm glad you're feeling better now and could make it to the party. UTIs can really knock you off your feet, can't they? Well, I have something that can change your mood.'

I immediately stood up, put on my best Rosesh Sarabhai voice and started reciting:

'Sit and ponder, without a care,

Toilet seats won't spread despair.

No need to fret, no need to stew,

Your bottom's fine, that much is true!'

She fake applauded as I took a seat next to her.

'*Kavi yeh kehna chahte hain ki* toilet seats do not cause infections!'[1]

She looked surprised as I kept talking.

Almost all disease-causing organisms[2] in urine are unable to survive outside the body or on hard surfaces and cannot be transmitted through skin contact with your bottom. The most common offender is Escherichia coli (E. coli), responsible for the majority of urinary tract infections (UTIs).[3] Infections caused by Escherichia coli can lead to diseases such as UTIs and pneumonia.[4] Similarly, another type of bacteria called Klebsiella spp. can cause faecal contamination and result in pneumonia, UTIs and other illnesses.[5] Actually, a study found that door handles, taps and counters in public toilets are even worse[6] than toilet seats when it comes to harbouring germs. While organisms that cause UTIs aren't transmitted by toilet seats, these high-touch surfaces can be more contaminated and pose a greater risk of spreading bacteria.

'I've penned a little poem to shed some light on this. Let me share it with you . . .' I was just about to narrate something when Fatema screamed.

'STOOOOOP!'

It was my turn to stare at her wide-eyed as Fatema turned into Geet.

'*Aap jo yeh bolte hai, iske paise charge karte hain ya muft ka gyaan hai? Kyunki chillar nahi hai mere paas!*'

As ever, she outdid my jokes, like she would do back in our school days. The familiar grin on her face assured me that we had triumphed in our battle against pseudoscience for the day.

Pimple Popping Pitfalls

Why It's Not All Fun and Games

During the summer holidays, our house in Mumbai became a hub for visiting relatives from near and far. The holidays seemed to draw them in like magnets, and soon, our home was filled with the laughter and chatter of family members catching up on lost time.

It was a typical Saturday afternoon and the air was filled with anticipation as my cousin's family, consisting of my cousin Priyanka, her husband Rajiv and their teenage daughter Aarvi, had come over for a visit.

During the week, they were busy sightseeing in the city. On the weekend, I had planned a fun outing for the evening—a movie followed by dinner. We debated for a while at the breakfast table the kind of movie we should go for and finally settled on a family comedy playing at the cinema.

Soon, it was afternoon and we all started getting ready to leave.

While everyone was busy around the house, I noticed Aarvi trying to pop a pimple in the mirror.

'Oye, what are you up to?' I asked her.

Priyanka rushed to my side. 'Oh, it's just one pimple. What harm could it do?'

'Actually, popping pimples can do more harm than good,' I explained.

Pimples, also known as acne in medical terms, occur when pores become clogged with oil, dead skin cells and bacteria. Acne is influenced by various factors, including genetic predisposition, stress levels, androgens and increased perspiration, all contributing to its onset and/or severity.[1]

When you try to squeeze or pop them, you risk pushing bacteria deeper into the skin, leading to inflammation and potential scarring. Picking at your skin can also increase the risk of infection and cause the pimple to take even longer to heal.[2]

I said, 'The scars caused by pimple popping are dark and can make your face look patchy.'

I noticed Priyanka looking at Aarvi sheepishly. Priyanka's face had many such scars, which had lightened with age but were still clearly visible.

Aarvi, who had been listening intently, chimed in with a worried expression. 'Does that mean I shouldn't pop any of my pimples?'

I nodded reassuringly. 'That's right, Aarvi. It's best to leave your skin alone and let pimples heal naturally. And if the pimples persist for a long time, it is good to see a dermatologist for them.'

I added, 'And remember, pimples are a common occurrence during adolescence.[3] Like many other challenges in life, they will come and go. Your confidence shouldn't hinge on their presence or absence.'

Moreover, there are plenty of other ways to take care of your skin and prevent it breaking out, like washing your face regularly with a gentle cleanser, using non-comedogenic moisturizers and avoiding touching your face with dirty hands.[4]

Aarvi and Priyanka shared a smile. Priyanka touched her ears and whispered, 'Sorry,' as Aarvi hugged her and said, 'How about a deal, Ma? No more pimple-popping and no neglecting our skin!' She extended her hand, asking her mother to promise.

One by one, we both placed our hands on hers and made a pact—to treat our body's largest organ, our skin, just like we treat other organs, with the utmost care and attention.

Sip Happens

Why Daily Wine Won't Keep the Doctor Away!

Warning: *Reading this may induce a sudden aversion towards that evening glass of wine—proceed at your own risk!*

At every family gathering, there's always that one relative who swears by the miraculous power of sipping one glass of wine daily. Got a similar 'health secret' sage in your clan?

Time to embark on a mission to prove them wrong! Let the family drama commence.

Drinking one glass of wine daily does not have any positive effect on your cardiovascular health.[1]

On the contrary, wine is a hydro-alcoholic solution and can be extremely harmful to your overall bodily health.[2]

So, basically, there's zilch medical proof that downing wine every day makes it a health tonic. Cheers to toasting your health every night with a beverage that's more of a myth than a miracle!

You've just survived another day in the corporate jungle, dodging deadlines and navigating office politics like a pro. As you finally kick off those painful pumps and sink into the couch, there it is: the siren call of a chilled glass of wine, beckoning you like a mirage in the desert of responsibility. We all know how this story ends.

But before you reach for that corkscrew. . . let's pause for a sobering reality check.

While that glass of wine might feel like the ultimate stress-reliever, the truth is it's just a fleeting mirage in the desert of self-care.

On the contrary, perhaps it would help to consider the fact that consuming a single bottle of wine weekly is linked to a rise in the overall lifetime risk of cancer, akin to smoking ten cigarettes weekly for women and five for men.[3]

Consumption of wine also has toxic effects on your gut and immune system.[4]

Oops! Looks like red wine has beef with your pancreas[5] too.

Regular wine intake appears to negatively affect blood pressure, homocysteine levels and your stomach.[6]

If drinking a glass of wine every night is your way of saying 'check' to life in the game of chess, then guess who is being check-mated here?

Breaking the Calcium Ceiling?

Debunking the Menopausal Misconception

As I stepped into my aunt's cosy living room, the familiar scent of incense and chai enveloped me in a warm embrace. It was a rare moment of respite from the hustle and bustle of my daily routine as a doctor, and I relished the opportunity to catch up with my family.

However, as fate would have it, our tranquil reunion was soon interrupted by the arrival of an unexpected guest: a delivery from the local chemist, bearing a month's supply of calcium supplements for my dear aunt.

Curiosity piqued, I couldn't help but inquire about the contents of the mysterious package. 'Aunty,' I asked, peering over her shoulder, 'what's all this?'

With a sheepish smile, she turned to face me, clutching the bottle of supplements in her hand. 'Oh, Manan *beta*,' she replied, 'it's just some calcium tablets. You know, for my bones.'

Brows furrowed in confusion, I pressed further. 'But Aunty, why do you need calcium supplements? Are you experiencing any bone-related complaints?'

With a dismissive wave of her hand, she brushed off my concerns. 'Oh, nothing like that, beta. I've just reached menopause, and all the ladies in my kitty party circle swear by these supplements. They say it's a must for women my age.'

My heart sank at her words. Here was my dear aunt, blindly following the advice of 'society ladies' without a second thought. It was a scenario all too familiar in our culture, where hearsay often holds more sway than scientific evidence.

Taking a deep breath, I decided to gently steer the conversation in a more informed direction. 'Aunty,' I began, choosing my words carefully, 'while it's true that calcium is important for bone health, it is recommended to use calcium supplements only when dietary intake is inadequate.'[1]

According to studies, the effectiveness of using calcium and Vitamin D to prevent fractures in all postmenopausal women remains uncertain.[2] Simply increasing calcium intake to counteract bone loss from menopause or ageing may not suffice.[3]

As I spoke, I could see the scepticism in my aunt's eyes giving way to curiosity. Here was a chance to empower her with knowledge and steer her away from the pitfalls of uninformed decisions.

I said, 'Recent research has challenged the notion that all postmenopausal women require calcium supplements, highlighting the potential risks associated with their indiscriminate use, particularly in relation to heart health. It's not advisable to add any supplemental calcium to the diet without medical guidance.'[4]

Out of the blue, a brilliant idea struck me, and I couldn't contain my excitement—I let out a loud scream. 'Actually, Aunty, there's something even better for keeping those bones strong!'

Aunty looked at me questioningly.

I explained, 'Strength training! It's like weightlifting and resistance exercises. They're fantastic for preserving bone density, especially for women after menopause. Studies show that strength training is even more effective at preventing bone loss. Plus, it has other benefits like improving balance and posture.'[5]

Aunty was sceptical. 'Hmm, I've never really lifted weights before. Isn't that something only bodybuilders do?'

'Not at all! You can start with light weights or even just use one-litre bottles filled with water. It's all about building up gradually. And trust me, you'll feel stronger and more confident in no time!' I assured her.

'Alright, you've convinced me! I'll give it a try. But no promises about becoming a bodybuilder!' She laughed.

By now her expression had softened, replaced by a newfound sense of understanding. 'Thank you, beta,' she said, her voice tinged with gratitude. 'I will return these right away and also share what you told me with my kitty group.'

With that, a weight seemed to lift from the room, replaced by a sense of relief and enlightenment. At that moment, I realized the true power of education and advocacy, even within the confines of our family circle.

As I bid my aunt farewell, I couldn't help but smile. Perhaps, just perhaps, I had managed to plant a seed of doubt in her mind, one that would blossom into a newfound sense of empowerment and autonomy over her health.

And in a world where misinformation often reigned supreme, that was a victory worth celebrating.

Keto *Kahaani* and *Kalesh*

Laughing Away Dieting Delusions

D ecember was the ultimate month for reunions. Friends and cousins scattered across the globe would flock back to India, turning it into a month-long celebration. Our calendars brimmed with breakfast and dinner invitations, while afternoons were reserved for shopping sprees.

On a Sunday, I was at a delightful breakfast hosted by my childhood friend, Animesh. Despite the miles and years between us, we've managed to stay close.

As I weighed my options between a steaming bowl of homemade gajar ka halwa and some guilt-free sugar-free cupcakes, Ananya's unmistakable voice cut through the chatter. Ananya was our group's resident songbird, her unique voice being the highlight at our gatherings. Spotting me, she made her way over, but I could tell something was different.

I signalled that she should grab a plate and join me, but I was surprised when she declined.

'I've stumbled upon a diet that seems to have finally worked for me!' she exclaimed. 'I've only been at it for two weeks, but I can feel the difference. Can you see it?' She twirled around expectantly, but I regarded her sceptically.

I asked, 'What's the name of this diet that's causing you to pass up on this feast?'

'Keto diet,' she replied eagerly and added, 'I read a couple of books on it and then did some more research on the internet and here I am. I have read it is the fastest and best way to lose weight.'

As I settled into a cosy corner with my plate, I explained, 'You see, Ananya, there's no such thing as the ultimate weight-loss solution. Keto, at most, can be considered just one of the numerous diets designed to shed those extra pounds. Like any other dietary regimen, it has both benefits and drawbacks. It is always advisable to consult a good doctor or a nutritionist before starting any such diet.'

There is also significant debate regarding the practicality of adopting the ketogenic diet as a long-term lifestyle choice and how sustainable it is without any negative impact on health or overall quality of life.[1]

'It's surprising to hear you say that, considering all I've ever heard are the endless benefits of keto. It's like it has no downsides whatsoever, right?' Ananya refused to take my advice.

'Where shall I start?' I was genuinely confused. 'For starters, a ketogenic diet is challenging to sustain as a long-term lifestyle and is only temporarily effective for weight reduction.'[2]

Ananya grabbed a cup of black coffee while we continued our discussion.

The ketogenic diet isn't regarded as holistic or as an all-natural remedy. Like any substantial medical intervention, it can lead to complications.[3] Common side effects include dizziness, nausea, increased urination, bad breath, palpitations, fatigue, constipation and muscle pain.[4] It also leads to a significant increase in the levels of low-density lipoprotein cholesterol.[5]

Some of the short-term side effects that occur when starting the ketogenic diet are often dubbed as keto flu. These symptoms include fatigue, headache, dizziness, nausea, vomiting, constipation and reduced exercise tolerance. Long-term consequences are hepatic steatosis, kidney stones, hypoproteinemia and vitamin deficiency.[6]

'You know, I've seen so many people regain all the weight they lost after stopping their diet because it's just not sustainable in the long term. They often don't gradually wean off the diet, which makes the weight rebound even more likely,' I exclaimed.

'That doesn't sound good!' Worry laced Ananya's voice.

'Consult a reputable doctor or nutritionist who can determine what works best for your body. Don't rely on the Internet or WhatsApp forwards for health advice,' I advised and suddenly noticed my bowl was empty.

'I need a second helping,' I said and got up from the table.

'Get something for me as well, please!' Ananya's voice was unmistakable.

As I turned around to confirm her request, she added, 'Your lessons left a bitter taste —now I need something sweet to balance it out!'

I nodded in agreement and walked towards the food table with a smile on my face. Once again, the power of science had come to the rescue.

Skin in the Drink

Hydration Hoax Exposed

One weekend, I visited my friend Priya, who was getting married soon. As we sat in the living room discussing wedding preparations, her teenage cousin, Ananya, kept coming in frequently, bringing water for Priya to drink. Curious, I asked, 'Why so much water?'

Ananya replied, '*Bhaiya*, water is great for good skin, and that's the only thing I rely on for my skin. No other products for me. Keeping the skin hydrated is crucial for maintaining its health and preventing dryness and wrinkles.'

She added with a smile, 'Since Didi is getting married, I want her to shine on her big day, so I'm reminding her to drink water.'

'Well, it's great to see you taking care of your health, Ananya. But did you know that the idea of drinking water to hydrate the skin is actually a common misconception?'[1] I asked her.

Ananya's expression turned to puzzlement as she looked at me for clarification.

I nodded, understanding her confusion. 'Yes, staying hydrated is important for overall health, but when it comes to skin hydration, the amount of water you drink isn't the only factor at play. In fact, research has shown that drinking excessive amounts of water won't necessarily improve skin hydration.'[2]

Ananya frowned, clearly surprised by this revelation.

While drinking water is important for overall health, there are other factors that play a more significant role in skin hydration. For example, using moisturizers and hydrating skincare[3] products can help lock in moisture and prevent dryness. Additionally, maintaining a healthy diet rich in fruits and vegetables, which are high in water content, can also contribute to skin hydration.[4]

Ananya listened intently, absorbing the information like a sponge. With a concerned expression, she set her water bottle aside and inquired, 'What's your recommendation?'

I replied, 'It's all about finding the right balance and adopting a holistic approach to skincare. Drinking water is certainly a part of that, but it's not the sole solution.'

If you want to smooth out those wrinkles and perk up your skin, it boils down to moisturizing and living that healthy lifestyle.[5] Most importantly, add more fruits, veggies, whole grains, healthy fats and lean proteins to your diet.[6]

'Bottom line? Guzzle water for good health, but don't bank on it for a wrinkle-free face. And keep in mind, there's no universal skincare solution for everyone. It's always a smart move to consult a dermatologist for personalized advice.' I smiled and gulped down a glass of water.

Priya chimed in, 'I'm planning to shop for some skincare creams tomorrow from my favourite brand. And guess what? I have gift coupons and discount vouchers!'

She then turned to Ananya with a grin. 'Why don't you come along? Let's have a skincare sesh with some gossip while I show you how to take care of your skin the fun way.'

Under Pressure

Debunking the High Blood Pressure Stress Fable

One day, I got a WhatsApp message from my cousin Dheeraj: 'I won't be able to make it to the family dinner this weekend. We're planning a staycation at the Taj.' It was unusual for him, so I replied, trying not to pry, 'Hey, no worries! We'll miss you, though. Hope everything's alright. Give my regards to Maya.'

Dheeraj replied with a lengthy message, 'I've been dealing with high blood pressure for weeks. The workload has been piling up and so has the stress. Maya thought a break might help me relax and lower my blood pressure. With summer holidays approaching, we couldn't plan a trip, so we opted for a small staycation to unwind.'

It was evening, and I was on my way home with my driver at the wheel. I decided it was the perfect time to have this conversation. The traffic was too noisy for a voice call, so we continued our conversation through messages.

I started typing furiously, 'Bro, a staycation with Maya sounds fantastic. You should definitely go for it. But seriously, stress doesn't cause high blood pressure.'[1]

The notion that stress plays a role in hypertension development has been prevalent for years, yet experimental studies have found a lack of sufficient evidence to support this claim.[2] High blood pressure, or hypertension, is a complex disorder influenced by various factors such as genetics, environment and demographics, contributing to its prevalence.[3] While stress and anxiety can indeed lead to temporary spikes in blood pressure, they don't always result in sustained elevations. It's crucial to understand that there are two types of stress: acute stress and chronic stress.[4] Although both can prompt a rise in blood pressure, their long-term impacts vary.

'Thanks, bro!' I could feel Dheeraj heave a sigh of relief.

'Enjoy the staycation on the weekend. And then come see me sometime next week at the clinic. It is time for some lifestyle changes!'

'I feel a sense of relief, like a burden has been lifted. I'll give you a call next week and come over. Let's do this, bro!'

Even though we weren't on a video call, I could feel the change in Dheeraj's energy.

I could see the sun setting outside, but science was shining brightly in our lives.

Inhale and Exhale

The Hidden Hazards of Hookahs

The radio played '*Tera pyar pyar pyar, hookah bar*' (Bollywood song lyrics loosely translating to 'Your love is like a hookah bar'). We were on a road trip to Manali with friends and had stopped at a dhaba on the highway for lunch.

Arnav, my friend, was belting out the song as I lounged in the back seat, trying to catch a quick nap after a satisfying meal.

Suddenly, he piped up, 'Guys, let's go to a hookah bar. I've heard Delhi's got some fantastic ones. It'll be the perfect way to wrap up our trip before catching our return flights the day after.'

All the sleep I had managed to grab evaporated upon hearing his suggestion. I was jolted awake and responded, 'Bro, I get your love for adventures, but this is a whole new level.'

By then, the rest of our friends had gathered around and were intrigued by our discussion. I explained what had happened and continued with the reasoning behind my reaction.

A hookah user encounters many of the same toxic compounds and by-products as cigarette users.[1] However, the levels are much higher, increasing the potential risks to health.[2] The belief that it causes less harm compared to cigarettes is wrong.[3]

Another friend intervened, 'Oh, bhai! We only have it occasionally. *Usse kuch nahi hota*! We have done it before and it was so much fun. It's all about good vibes, having a blast and unwinding. Moreover, it even smells nice!'

'Oh, of course, once in a blue moon makes it totally justified, right?' I asked.

He nodded.

'WRONG!' I screamed, 'The disastrous effects of hookah are just too many to ignore. It's a time bomb waiting to go off.'

Hookah smoke contains significant quantities of carcinogenic substances like hydrocarbons and heavy metals.[4] It contains higher levels of harmful substances compared to cigarettes. A regular hookah smoker's blood nicotine levels are equivalent to those of a cigarette smoker who smokes ten cigarettes a day.[5] Moreover, hookahs are also offered in flavours that appeal particularly to young people. They are marketed as harmless and tasty. However, the reality is quite different.

Their widened eyes told me I had to see this through to the end.

'I know this might feel like one of the episodes of *Darna Mana Hai*, but it isn't. *Darna zaruri hai*, bro!' I paused for effect before continuing, 'From your lungs to your heart, from weight gain to your pearly whites, it's got the power to wreck it all.'

Hookah smoking is associated with a higher risk of obesity.[6] It is also known to create complications with heart rate and blood pressure along with other cardiovascular issues.[7] COPD and other lung-related ailments are also some of the ill effects of hookah consumption.[8]

The silence was shattered by Harsh's voice cutting through it like a knife through butter. 'I always thought those hookah joints were harmless hangouts.'

'Well, now you know, they are not!' I put my hand on the shoulder of Arnav, who was sitting in the front, and said, 'Bro, I know love is blind, but not blind enough to fall for a hookah bar!'

Right then, the radio decided to serenade us with '*Kar de mushkil jeena, ishq kameena*' (Bollywood lyrics translating to 'This love is a rascal as it makes it difficult to live'), reminding us that love, in all its quirky forms, isn't exactly a cakewalk. But we still choose it, unlike a hookah bar!

Flexing the Truth

Debunking the Creatine Conundrum

As I settled into a cosy corner of our favourite cafe, surrounded by the familiar faces of old friends, I couldn't help but relish the opportunity to catch up on the latest gossip and laughs.

'So, peeps,' my friend Aarohi declared, her tone tinged with exasperation, 'I finally decided to quit my gym membership. Turns out, they were making me take creatine supplements, and I swear it made my hair fall out!'

'Well, good thing you're not taking them anymore,' another friend, Rahul, chimed in with a mischievous grin. 'I've heard creatine causes all sorts of, ahem, performance issues *downstairs*.'

The table erupted with laughter at Rahul's cheeky remark, but beneath the jests, I sensed a hint of genuine concern. It was time to set the record straight and debunk these gym-related myths once and for all.

'Actually,' I interjected, my voice laced with sincerity, 'there's a lot of misinformation out there about creatine. Contrary to popular belief, it's one of the safest and most researched supplements out there.'[1]

Creatine is a naturally occurring compound found in our muscles. Taking a small dose of around 5 grams per day can actually enhance athletic performance, increase muscle mass and improve strength.[2]

Most creatine-rich foods are animal products.[3] And can you imagine how many sunflower seeds you would need to eat daily to meet your creatine needs?

Taking creatine supplements alongside resistance training can boost both maximum strength and endurance as well as muscle growth.[4]

Regardless of gender and age, creatine can be taken in the recommended amount. It has beneficial effects on strength, power, lean muscle mass, daily functioning and neurological function in both young and older individuals.[5]

The table fell silent as my friends absorbed this newfound knowledge, their eyes wide with wonder. Here was a chance to dispel the myths and misconceptions surrounding supplements and to empower them with the truth.

Research suggests that creatine does not cause hair loss, erectile dysfunction or kidney damage.[6]

'As for hair loss and . . . well, you know,' I chuckled, 'it's like believing in ghosts—great for a scare, but not grounded in reality!'

Carbonated Comedy

The Bubbly Truth About Soft Drinks

O ne afternoon, while on a shopping spree with my friend Saahil, we decided to seek refuge in a nearby restaurant. Eager to quench his thirst, Saahil promptly ordered a soft drink and a sandwich, while I ordered a masala dosa and sugar-less coffee.

The soft drink was the first to be served in a can, as requested by Saahil. As soon as the waiter left, I couldn't help but raise an eyebrow at his choice.

'Soft drinks? Seriously?' I exclaimed, unable to contain my surprise.

Saahil shrugged casually. 'Hey, I know they are high in sugar, but it's okay to indulge once in a while, right?' he replied, popping open his can with a satisfying hiss.

I shook my head in disbelief. 'Actually, no, it's not okay,' I retorted. 'And it's not just because of the high sugar content. Soft drinks, or aerated drinks, as they're often called, are horrendously unhealthy. They are empty calories with no nutritional value.'

Saahil looked puzzled. 'But they're so refreshing and everyone drinks them,' he protested.

Just then, my dosa and coffee arrived along with Saahil's sandwich. I took a bite of my dosa and leaned forward, adopting a serious tone. 'Well, if we're applying that logic, we might as well start justifying every addiction under the sun, right?'

Drinking soft drinks can have negative effects on both oral and overall health.[1] Research has shown time and again that regular consumption of soft drinks is linked to a host of health problems, including obesity, type 2 diabetes[2] and tooth decay.[3] In some extreme cases, soft drinks are also linked to tooth loss due to dental decay or gum diseases.[4]

Soft drinks deplete calcium from the body, leading to an excess amount of calcium that tends to accumulate in the kidneys, resulting in kidney stone formation. I looked him right in the eye and said, 'In short, soft drinks should come with a warning label akin to those on cigarette packs: "IT IS INJURIOUS TO HEALTH".'[5]

Saahil looked confused. 'Yaar, what does this leave me with?' By now, he had put his soft drink aside after having a few sips.

I grinned, relieved that he was open to making a change. 'Water is always a safe bet,' I suggested. 'It's refreshing, hydrating and has zero calories. Plus, you can always add a splash of lemon or a few mint leaves for some extra flavour.'

Just then, I spotted a coconut vendor outside the restaurant and said, 'Or we can also have fresh coconut water.'

'Well, those seem like a wild ride for me, considering I've been riding the sugar rollercoaster all these years!' Saahil laughed and joined me on a new adventure.

Mind over Myth

Breaking Down Mental Health Misconceptions

The aroma of freshly brewed coffee was in the air when Sunita Masi and her husband Ajay Masa came home one Sunday morning. Their son Mayank was getting married soon and they had come to invite us to the wedding.

As we settled down in the cosy living room, the conversation flowed freely, touching upon everything from work and family to politics and current events.

But amid the light-hearted banter, there was a momentary lull in the conversation as my father inquired about Rahul Mama, who was battling mental health issues.

Masi mentioned his recent struggles and remarked, 'It's such a shame about poor Rahul,' while wiping her tears.

'But I suppose a mental health condition is just a sign of weakness, isn't it? If he were stronger, he wouldn't be in this situation,' Ajay Masa added with a sympathetic shake of his head.

Their words hung in the air, met with a mixture of discomfort and uncertainty from the rest of us. But I didn't want that statement to go unchallenged.

'Masa, mental health conditions are not a sign of weakness at all,' I interjected, my voice calm yet firm. 'They are mental conditions, just like any other illness, and can affect anyone regardless of their strength or character.'[1]

As I spoke, I could see the surprise and curiosity in Sunita Masi's eyes as well as in those of the others, prompting me to delve deeper into the topic.

'Mental health issues can arise due to a variety of factors, including genetic predisposition, environmental stressors and chemical imbalances in the brain,' I continued, my tone earnest. 'And it's important to recognize that seeking support and treatment are not signs of weakness, but rather signs of strength and courage.[2] Nowadays, we have expert help readily available for any mental health–related issues. From psychiatrists and psychologists to therapists and counsellors, there are professionals who can assist those struggling with mental health challenges to lead better lives. Seeking therapy or consulting a psychiatrist is no longer taboo. In fact, it should be appreciated and encouraged when someone takes that step (learn more about therapy on page 180).'

As I spoke, I could see Sunita Masi nodding along thoughtfully, her initial scepticism giving way to an understanding and empathy for those struggling with mental health issues.

'By breaking down the barriers and misconceptions surrounding mental health, we can create a more inclusive and supportive environment in which individuals feel empowered to seek help without fear of judgement or discrimination,' I explained. 'And by fostering open and honest conversations about mental health, we can work together to ensure that everyone has access to the care and support they need to live happy, healthy and fulfilling lives.'[3]

Sunita Masi looked at me teary-eyed when I said, 'I believe it's okay if we're unable to directly assist Rahul Mama, but speaking about his mental health in such a manner isn't appropriate. It's crucial to acknowledge and respect the difficulties he's facing and extend our support in any possible way.'

She stood up and embraced me, remarking, 'Who says only elders impart wisdom to children? Sometimes, elders learn valuable lessons from kids too. Thank you, Manan beta. This has been quite an eye-opener.'

Detox Decoded

Unmasking the Grand Illusion

Eight out of ten products you see today on a supermarket aisle have 'detox' screaming from their packaging. And let's not forget the kaleidoscope of colours in the detox market. From green juices that promise to turn you into the Hulk (minus the green complexion) to charcoal-infused concoctions that claim to absorb toxins like a black hole, it's a carnival! Is it or is it not?

Detox is basically a process in which the body is cleaned and all the toxins removed. If you study them closely, all the detox products help you get rid of something from your body. They call this process 'flushing out' and the list of things they can help you get rid of includes toxins and fat, among others.

One might not be able to trace the origin of the detox culture, but we all do remember the promises they made of shedding toxins, revitalizing energies and sipping on herbal elixirs.

Pick any popular detox product and its cover reads, '*Flush out the toxins . . . !*' in one way or another.

Have you ever wondered where? Is there a secret route in your body, unknown to you, that is aiding this process?

Let's find out.

Nature has equipped our bodies to naturally flush out toxins and any other unwanted waste on their own. This process involves the liver, kidneys, skin, lungs and digestive system. Toxins leave our body the same way they enter—through our breath, sweat, urine, gut and bowels. There are no other secret gates in our body for this process.

Expecting detox to cleanse our body is like expecting a plant to thrive on soda instead of water—it's a novel idea, but Mother Nature disagrees.

So are all the detox plans and products useless?

Well, yes. Medically speaking, detox is a delusion.[1]

Moreover, there is little evidence to prove the impact of detox diets on health.[2] Irrespective of the duration for which these detox products or diets have been followed, they have no substantial effect on weight loss or weight management.[3]

Detox tea is an illusion that keeps on giving (do read **Spill the Tea** to know more about it).

So the next time someone pitches a detox miracle, RUNNNN... It's a trap! Because your body has been acing the detox game without relying on enchanted teas or mysterious rituals.

Pour Decisions

Rinsing Away the Mealtime Water Delusion

onfession Time: Do you belong to the team that sips water before, after and during meals or the one that steers clear of it before, after or during meals?

Count me in the first category, and I've got plenty of good reasons to back that choice. How about you?

Let us take the lead and explain the reasons.

Drinking water before, after and during a meal is absolutely safe and harmless.[1] Water is essential for every living being. The human body's composition of water ranges from 75 per cent in infants to 55 per cent in the elderly, playing a crucial role in cellular homeostasis and sustaining life.[2]

If your body is signalling you to drink water, it means there is a water deficit in your body, making you thirsty.[3] On the contrary, not drinking enough water at such a time could lead to disastrous effects on physiological and psychological health.

Our health can be compromised if deficits in body water result in significant disruptions to the body's water balance.[4] Body water balance is the net difference between water gain and water loss.

So how much water should you drink? Well, science has not been able to find an answer to this.[5] Despite countless attempts to unveil this magical number, it seems the universal answer remains hidden in the dark cosmos.

However, staying hydrated is always beneficial. Don't stress too much about those frequent bathroom trips after hydrating. Your kidneys are just showing off their skills! Moreover, the colour of your urine, ranging from pale yellow to clear, serves as a reliable gauge of hydration levels.

From aiding in cellular functions to the digestion process and from improving concentration to making the skin glow due to hydration,[6] this wondrous elixir is the key to all.

If you are still confused about which team to be a part of, then it might be high time to break the bridge and forge a new path.

And for Team Sip-Sip, the next time someone tries to stop you from sipping water between bites, just wink and tell them it's your secret sauce for smoother chewing!

Spot On

Embracing the Quirks
of Your Skin

I adore my gym time. Besides helping me sculpt my body, it's my escape from the mundane. I thrive on the adrenaline rush my workouts bring.

A few weeks back, as I was finishing up my session, I overheard two young girls chatting in the gym. It was getting late and the music had stopped for reasons only the admins knew. The conversation, which was being carried out in low voices, could be heard quite clearly.

Soon, I found out that one of them, G1, was getting married in a few months and was fretting over dark patches on her intimate areas, elbows and knees. The other, G2, suggested skin-lightening treatments.

G2 shared, 'I was in this position a few weeks ago when a relative suggested skin-lightening treatment to my mother.'

G1 said, 'I wanted to ask you the same thing. I wanted your opinion on this and if you know someone reliable.'

As they discussed the cost, I couldn't help but intervene: 'Sorry to interrupt, but I'm Manan, a qualified doctor. I couldn't help overhearing your conversation and wanted to share some medical insights. If you don't mind?'

After they agreed, I had a heart-to-heart with the two ladies. ' Look, I understand your concern, but dark patches on the skin, particularly in those areas, are quite common[1] and usually nothing[2] to be concerned about.'

G1's expression softened with relief as she listened attentively to my explanation. 'Really? But what could be causing them?'

I took a moment to gather my thoughts before responding. 'Well, the skin in certain areas of our body, like the groin, underarms, knees and elbows, naturally tends to be darker due to factors like friction, hormonal changes and even genetics. In the case of the private areas, the skin is naturally darker to provide and maintain moisture levels.[3] So it's completely normal to notice some variation in skin tone in these regions.'

G2 nodded thoughtfully, seeming to absorb the information. 'I see. That does make sense. But is there anything we can do to lighten the patches?'

I chuckled softly, realizing that both of them were still contemplating remedies. 'Honestly, there's no need to worry about lightening these areas. Trying to alter the natural pigmentation of the skin can often do more harm than good. Instead, it's important to focus on maintaining good hygiene and overall skin health.'

If dark skin patches in areas like the back of the neck, armpits and groin appearing as velvety, hyperpigmented patches with unclear boundaries, then it is a medical concern. It is known as Acanthosis nigricans, which is often linked to diabetes and insulin resistance. It is recommended to seek medical guidance in this case.[4]

G1 seemed to relax further, visibly relieved by my reassurance. 'Thank you so much for explaining, Dr Manan. I feel much better now knowing that it's nothing serious.'

I looked at them and said, 'Each of us is unique in countless ways; our skin tone, eye colour, height, weight, hair colour—all of these traits make us who we are. I understand that the market is filled with quick "fixes" that take advantage of insecurities and promise fairness or slimness or height. Ignore all that noise and celebrate this special occasion. Don't let such things bother you. A wedding is a beautiful occasion. Just focus on the preparations, the beautiful clothes, the delicious sweets to be made, the songs to dance to—and the fun you will all have together.'

Both the girls looked at me teary-eyed and nodded while mouthing 'thank you'!

Smoke Signals

The Comedy of Smoking Conundrums

As I strolled down the bustling streets of Mumbai, the familiar scent of chai and the distant hum of traffic filled the air. It was just another day in the city of dreams and I was on my way to catch up with a friend.

Spotting him from across the street, I quickened my pace, eager to catch up after what felt like ages. But as I drew closer, I saw my friend, Ashish, leaning against a lamp post with a cigarette dangling from his lips.

'Ashish!' I exclaimed, unable to mask my shock. 'When did you start smoking?'

With a sheepish grin, he shrugged nonchalantly. 'Oh, just a little stress relief, Manan. Nothing to worry about.'

But I knew better than to dismiss his words so easily. 'Stress relief, huh? And how's that working out for you?' I countered, my voice laced with concern.

Ashish waved away my question with a dismissive gesture. 'Oh, you know how it is, Manan. Just a couple of cigarettes a day, nothing too serious. Once this project at work is over, I'll quit for good.'

'Does your boss know he is the reason behind you picking up this new habit?' I asked, trying hard to not sound angry.

Ashish looked at me questioningly.

I explained, 'Just curious, you see!'

As Ashish puffed away some smoke rings, I could imagine him mentally swearing at my bad jokes. But I knew this wasn't a joke and so I started waving the red flag through my words for him to notice.

'Ashish, my friend,' I began, my words tinged with urgency, 'smoking is no joke. Whether you smoke two cigarettes a day or twenty, the damage to your health is irreversible.'

Smoking cigarettes is considered a significant risk factor for the onset of lung cancer. On average, smokers have a reduced lifespan of around eight years. Tobacco is the leading cause of adult mortality in developed nations. Cigarette smoking, along with other risk factors like high blood pressure and high cholesterol, can lead to the development and worsening of clogged arteries.[1]

Smokers experience decreased fertility.[2] Tobacco smoking leads to widespread death and disability.[3] The main reason is that cigarettes quickly deliver nicotine to the brain in an easy-to-consume and enjoyable form. Nicotine affects the brain by triggering cravings to smoke in situations where smoking is common and when nicotine levels in the brain drop.[4]

After what felt like an eternity of heartfelt conversation, Rohan finally relented, extinguishing his cigarette with a determined flick of his wrist.

'You may be right, Manan, but I will also be honest here,' he admitted, his voice tinged with resolve. 'I am sure you know that it is not possible to stop smoking overnight, but I will gradually try to reduce my cigarette consumption.'

'That's a great decision! It's no walk in the park, but hang in there. Be patient and don't throw in the towel halfway. If needed, consult a de-addiction specialist to help you kick the smoking habit for good.'

Dialling Down the Drama

Why Sleeping with Your Phone Is A-Okay!

O nce annually, our crew of cousins embarks on a trip. With some of us grown up and others still in their teens, it's a fantastic opportunity to strengthen our bond. We select a destination and meticulously plan for months leading up to the journey. This year, we settled on the mountains and found ourselves in Manali. The stunning peaks, clear blue skies, fresh air and endless laughter made the trip absolutely delightful.

One evening, the sun was setting, casting a warm glow over our tired faces as my cousins and I returned to our cosy cottage after a long day of hiking during our trip. Eager to rest our weary bodies, we began to settle in for the night when suddenly, chaos ensued.

One of my cousins, Riya, exclaimed, her voice alarmed, 'Kartik, what are you doing? How many times do I have to tell you that's bad for your health?'

Intrigued by Riya's outburst, I couldn't help but inquire further. 'What's the matter, Riya? Why is sleeping with a phone under the pillow such a big deal?'

Riya turned to me with a look of grave concern. 'Well, Manan,' she began, her tone sombre, 'sleeping with your phone nearby can disrupt your sleep patterns, mess with your brain waves and even increase your risk of cancer!'

Suppressing a poorly timed yawn, I decided it was time to set the record straight. 'Actually, Riya, that's just a common misconception,' I said, drawing upon my medical knowledge. 'There's no scientific evidence[1] to support those claims. In fact, radio frequency radiation, a type of electromagnetic radiation emitted by phones, is so low that it poses no significant risk[2] to our health.'

Kartik, who had been listening intently, nodded in agreement. 'Yeah, Riya, I think you might be overreacting a bit. I've been sleeping with my phone nearby for years and I've never had any issues.'

I nodded in solidarity with Kartik. 'Exactly! As long as we're using our phones responsibly[3] and practising good sleep hygiene, there's no reason to panic.'

Riya still seemed sceptical, so I decided to offer some reassurance based on my expertise. 'You see, Riya,' I explained, 'our phones emit non-ionizing radiation,[4] which is different from the ionizing radiation[5] that can cause harm. The levels of radiation from our phones are simply too low to cause any health problems.'[6]

The human body absorbs energy from devices emitting radio frequency radiation.[7] The only widely acknowledged biological effect of this absorption is heating in the area of the body where a cell phone is held, such as the ear and the head. However, this heat isn't enough to significantly raise core body temperature.[8] No other harmful health effects from radio frequency radiation[9] on the human body have been clearly established.

The reasons why people worry that cell phones could lead to certain types of cancer or other health issues[10] are understandable. However, the current evidence indicates that cell phone use does not lead to brain or other types of cancer in humans.[11]

The frequency of radio frequency radiation from a mobile phone is low and is less than 8 Ghz.[12] According to studies, low-level RF fields above 6 GHz are not harmful to human health.[13]

Riya's expression softened as she processed this information. 'Wow, I had no idea,' she admitted sheepishly. 'I guess I got caught up in all the fear-mongering.'

'Furthermore, keeping your phone (on silent mode to avoid disturbance while sleeping) nearby ensures sweet dreams, courtesy of all the love and kisses in the messages,' I teased with a wink.

Upon hearing this, Riya hurled a pillow at me, shouting, 'Manan!' and soon our AirBnB accommodation had turned into a war zone as pillow fights ensued.

Whey's Up?

Liver and Kidney Tales Exposed!

One weekend, during a small, intimate get-together, our conversation naturally drifted towards fitness and gym routines. As we shared our various gym stories, Prachi, a relatively new member of our friends' circle, hesitantly voiced her concerns.

'I've heard that consuming whey protein is essential when you're gymming,' she began, her eyes reflecting genuine worry. 'But I've also heard it's not good for your health. Is that true? Are all of you using whey protein? And what about its side effects?'

We all paused, sensing her apprehension.

'Why? What's wrong with whey protein?' I needed answers.

She clarified, 'Manan, you are a doctor. Of all people, you should know that whey protein can damage the liver and kidneys. It is not safe to consume.'

'No, Prachi,' I shook my head. 'Whey protein is completely safe for consumption.'

Before anyone could answer, I jumped in to reassure her.

'Did you know, depending on the stage of lactation, breast milk contains 50-80 per cent whey protein?[1] So, technically, we've all had it before!' I said, smiling.

'Really?' she asked, looking surprised.

'Yes, absolutely,' I continued. 'It's totally safe. As long as you have a healthy liver and kidneys, you can consume whey protein without any worries.'

Whey is a component of milk and a co-product of cheese-making and casein manufacture in the dairy industry. This makes it a completely natural product.[2]

Actually, the perks of whey are too numerous to tally up! Bioactive compounds in whey fight off germs, boost the immune system, strengthen bones and protect against cancer and heart disease.[3] They also enhance the quick recovery of exercise performance following intense resistance training.[4]

'And if I'm not mistaken, you're a vegetarian, right?' I asked, looking at Prachi. She nodded in agreement.

'All the more reason whey protein is recommended for you, because it can be quite challenging for vegetarians to meet their daily protein needs,'[5] I explained.

Research indicates that reaching and sustaining a healthy weight can extend your lifespan and keep away weight-related issues such as diabetes, cancer and heart disease.[6]

The best part is that it is highly absorbent. The body easily absorbs the whey protein without any digestion issues.[7]

With every line I said, the expressions on everyone's faces changed from shock to surprise to, finally, acknowledgment.

I grabbed a glass of water kept on the table and gulped it down in one go. Finally, I took a deep breath and said in my best Kareena Kapoor imitation, '*Aap* convince *ho gaye, ya main aur bolu?*'

Spill the Tea

Myth: Green tea is good for weight loss.

Knock knock.
Who's there?
Green tea!
Green tea who?
Green tea who makes you lose weight.

Type these seven words into your Google search bar and you will see a plethora of results recommending various brands and types of teas to achieve this. How true are they?

Let's explore. Originating in China, tea made from unfermented leaves is called green tea. Though its name suggests that it is, it may or may not be green in colour. The shades range from light brown to liquid gold. Tea is a huge part of South Asian culture. Various types of tea are flooding the market, including green tea, white tea, yellow tea and blue tea. Each one claims to have a list of benefits longer than the other.

Contrary to the traditional method of boiling fermented tea leaves in water with milk and sugar, green tea preparation does not include boiling the unfermented leaves with water. The process is known as steeping—the leaves are added only after the water has started boiling and the gas has been turned off. The unfermented leaves are considered to be very delicate and any over-cooking can ruin their fine flavours. Unlike the popular version of tea leaves cooked with milk and sugar, green tea is slightly bitter in taste and is consumed without milk and sugar (in most cases!).

This tea is 99.9 per cent water and is largely devoid of any nutrients or calories. It is different from regular tea and yet is similar. They have a common ingredient called caffeine, which increases your alertness and performance. With these benefits echoing across social media platforms today, everyone is advocating for these versions of milk-less, sugar-less teas.

So is green tea good for weight loss?

No, green tea has no significant impact on weight loss.[1]

But it is still good, right? After all, what harm can flavoured hot water cause?

Wrong. Consumption of green tea for a long time may result in increased hunger and decreased thirst.[2] Higher intake of green tea can also impact the liver adversely.[3]

The recommended dose of green tea is three to five cups a day.[4]

Anything in excess, even the most beneficial practices, can turn from elixir to poison for our well-being. Just like a balanced diet and regular exercise, moderation is key. Embrace a balanced lifestyle for lasting health.

Before you break up with your green tea squad, hold on a sec. Turns out, this leafy potion has a few tricks up its sleeve. It's the Houdini of beverages. Who knew?

Regular consumption of green tea does have some benefits, such as lowering your risk of cardiovascular diseases.[5] However, it has no impact on one's weight. Green tea is to weight loss what egg yolk is to cholesterol—a mythical tale without scientific grounding (confused? Read 'Cracking the Egg Joke' on page 286 to know more).

Crunching in the Dark

Shedding Light on Late-Night Snack Shenanigans

A reunion of childhood friends in the mountains. Sounds idyllic, right?

Late-night heart-to-hearts, leisurely strolls in nature's embrace, attempting to whip up some Maggi in the AirBnB we'd booked like we used to do at the hostel—the past three days had felt like a journey back in time.

Since we were leaving the next day, we made a pact to stay up all night and talk. Like the good old days when our exams were over and we were heading home the next day.

We were engrossed in laughter and conversation when Kashyap gestured for us to take notice of Imran, who seemed lost in thought. Assuming he was preoccupied with his upcoming wedding, as he was soon to be married, we all began teasing him relentlessly.

'Arre yaar! It's nothing like that. The thing is, my gym instructor advised against midnight snacking, but I'm feeling really hungry!' He sounded annoyed.

Ashish added, 'I am hungry too!'

Within seconds, the atmosphere in the room had shifted. The jovial faces that were laughing and joking a few minutes ago now appeared hungry and confused.

'Bro, what's with the confusion? We can just grab a bite right now. Let me see what options we have,' I said.

As I rose from my seat, heading towards the room where my bags were, they screamed together, 'Come on, Manan, you're a doctor. You're supposed to stop us when we suggest things that are bad for our health, not encourage our foolishness like this.'

'But what you suggested isn't bad for health![1] What matter are food choices and portion size.'

While there's no denying that overindulging in heavy, calorie-laden meals before bedtime can disrupt sleep and contribute to weight gain,[2] it's important to recognize that not all late-night snacks are created equal. A light, balanced snack containing protein and healthy fats can actually be beneficial.[3]

'I would have stopped you if you wanted to have a high-calorie meal,' I added, sitting down next to them with my bag.

'Foods like Greek yoghurt, nuts or a small serving of fruit can help stabilize blood sugar levels and promote better sleep quality,'[4] I said, taking out a packet of nuts and a bagful of oranges I had bought that day.

With every item that came out of my bag, their expressions changed from surprise to amazement to sheer joy.

Kashyap was the first to get up. 'I have an old newspaper we can use to spread out our snacks.' Imran was next, 'I will bring a bag to gather all the waste. Once we're settled, Ashish, you need to continue your story about Neha, your new colleague and crush.' He emphasized the word 'crush' with air quotes and continued, 'I got distracted by hunger, but now I'm back and eager to know what happened next.'

Amid oohs and aahs, we cracked some tough nuts and delved into the mystery of Ashish's love life.

I am sharing a secret with you, dear readers—all his previous crushes existed only in his imagination!

BMI

Bizarre Metrics Inside

I n today's modern era, technology serves as both a blessing and a curse. While it has significantly shrunk the world and facilitated seamless connectivity, it has also proliferated fake information, misleading forwarded messages and general chaos, particularly in the realm of health and medicine.

The number of WhatsApp groups I am a part of must be double my age, and some I can't even recall joining. Typically, I simply ignore them as they're often on mute. However, today was an exception. I had to attend a conference in Pune and had booked a cab for a late-night return to Mumbai. As the driver chauffeured me to my destination, I leisurely scrolled through messages on my phone.

One of my many WhatsApp group chats pinged with a new message. I couldn't help but chuckle at the screenshot someone had shared. It was their BMI score along with a proud declaration that they were in the 'normal' range.

'Hey folks, check out my BMI! Looks like I'm right on track for a healthy body!' the message read.

I couldn't resist the urge to intervene. After all, as a doctor, it's practically my duty to bust such myths. So I typed out my response, hoping to inject some truth into the conversation.

'Hey, I hate to burst your bubble, but BMI is so last decade! It's time we embraced a more accurate measure of fitness and body size: body composition.'[1]

Almost immediately, the group erupted with curious responses, eager to learn more about this newfangled concept I was preaching.

'But Dr Manan, isn't BMI the gold standard for measuring health?' one member questioned.

I chuckled at the outdated notion. 'Not anymore, my friend! BMI, or body mass index, is a relic from a bygone era. It's a simple calculation based solely on height and weight, and it doesn't take into account factors like muscle mass or fat distribution.'[2]

Another member chimed in, 'But isn't a lower BMI better for your health?'

I shook my head, amused by the widespread misunderstanding. 'Not necessarily! A low BMI is not always a positive and a high BMI is not a negative. It can be misleading, especially for individuals with higher muscle mass. They might have a higher BMI due to their muscle weight, but that doesn't mean they're unhealthy.'

I took a moment to compose my thoughts before continuing. 'That's where body composition comes in. Unlike BMI, which only considers weight relative to height, body composition provides a more detailed breakdown of your body's composition including muscle mass, fat percentage and bone density.'[3]

Body composition plays a vital role in maintaining overall health and longevity. It's influenced by various factors such as genetics, environment and lifestyle choices. Assessing body composition is crucial as it helps effectively evaluate nutritional status.[4]

You can get a detailed report on body composition as part of a DEXA Body Scan[5] conducted by a DXA machine at any radiology clinic. This is the most accurate way to do the body composition analysis.

'So what should we focus on instead of BMI?' someone asked eagerly.

'Simple!' I replied with a grin emoji, 'Focus on building muscle, reducing body fat and maintaining a balanced diet and exercise routine. By prioritizing healthy habits and tracking your body composition, you'll get a much clearer picture of your overall health and fitness.'

'Sounds so easy, bro!' One group member sent this message with a winking face emoji.

The number of laughing emoticons that followed this was proof enough that science had once again come to the rescue!

The Label Fable

Adventures in Food Fiction

L ast month, I had an intriguing patient visit my clinic—Pankaj Patel, a cheerful and straightforward man in his early forties. A few months ago, Panjakbhai had been diagnosed with borderline diabetes and high cholesterol. He sought our consultation after feeling dissatisfied with his previous doctor. The test results were alarming, showing a deterioration from bad to worse. During my routine inquiries about his dietary habits—what he ate, when and how much—a particular phrase caught my attention: 'I consume only fat-free items.' From snacks to sugar-free chocolates and cookies, he opted exclusively for fat-free foods.

The term 'fat-free' began to echo like a broken record in my mind as I attempted to connect his lab results with this revelation.

I gestured for him to take a seat and set his file aside. As he settled in and sipped some water, I delivered the news: 'It seems your perspective on food might need a little correction.'

Many food labels are deceptive,[1] including those claiming to be healthy, organic, immune-boosting and fat-free. Food labels serve as a marketing tactic[2] as well. Items that are low or devoid of one component often contain a high amount of another.[3] Food labelling can impact consumers' perception of food quality and influence their dietary choices.[4]

Let me tell you about an interesting study, where they found that easy-to-understand front labels on products encouraged companies to change their ingredients. In contrast, labels with only numerical data, without specific guidance, had little impact on reducing unhealthy nutrients. The most common outcomes were sodium, sugar and calorie reduction.[5]

'Are you saying they lied to me?' Pankajbhai asked in a heavy Gujarati accent.

'It is marketing, Pankajbhai. It's not just about the labels; there's a whole array of factors influencing consumer decisions,[6] from the packaging colour, name and font to the images on the packet, among other elements.'

Research suggests that the labels on food items can pull quite the magic trick on consumers. They can make you believe that you're reaching for the healthiest option while simultaneously preparing your taste buds for disappointment.[7]

Green-coloured packaging is considered healthier while ticks and seals are considered signs of authenticity.[8] 'Natural ingredients only' and 'free from artificial colours and flavours' are attractive attributes[9] that hold no truth. Technically, they are nothing but wordplay. Calling a jelly fat-free is like calling seawater sugar-free!

While dancing around with enticing health claims, these food labels are like sneaky magicians, convincing you that you're making the healthiest choice, all while leading you into a taste bud trap![10]

'Arre, Pankajbhai. Leave the labels or they will leave you singing, "*Dus bahane karke de gayi* bill" (popular Hindi song translating to "After giving ten excuses, she handed you the bill")!'

'*Ae no hale*, Mananbhai!' Pankajbhai laughed.

Shortly afterwards, I reached out to the nutritionist, and together we revamped his dietary habits. Just another day, just another life saved by science.

Lifting Lightweights

Why Kids in the Gym Shouldn't Be a Heavy Concern

One Sunday morning, as the sun peeked through my window, I was greeted by the ringing of my phone. Groggily, I picked it up to find my cousin Mohit on the other end, sounding distressed.

'Manan bhai, Ma is really angry with me,' he blurted out, his voice urgent with worry.

'What happened, Mohit?' I asked, concern creeping into my voice as I heard his mother's scolding in the background.

'I told Ma I wanted to join the gym in my summer holidays and she flipped out,' he explained. 'I mentioned that you suggested it to me and now she wants to talk to you.'

Mamta Kaki's overprotective instincts were legendary in the family, but I hadn't expected this extreme reaction. Mohit, barely a teenager, had recently expressed interest in fitness during a family gathering. Sensing an opportunity for him to stay active and healthy while focusing on his studies, I had casually suggested he take up gymming during his summer break.

Taking a deep breath, I instructed Mohit to pass the phone to his mother. 'Hello, Mamta Kaki,' I greeted her warmly, mentally preparing myself for the impending conversation.

'Manan, I did not expect this from you. Being an elder brother, you should guide him on the right path. How could you suggest something so risky to Mohit?' Kaki was fuming.

After listening to her concerns, I calmly explained, 'Kaki, gymming knows no age limits. Regardless of age, everyone can and should engage in physical activity suitable for their capacity.'

'But Manan,' Mamta Kaki interrupted me and added, 'I am worried about his height. As it is, he is shorter than the others in his class. I have heard that working out in the gym at such a young age can impact his height.' She sounded concerned.

'This is not true at all, Kaki,' I explained.

Engaging in physical exercise doesn't hinder a child's growth or development. Instead, it plays a role in shaping bones and muscle tissues. It also offers potential benefits throughout their life.[1]

Physical exercise is a planned and repetitive activity aimed at improving or maintaining your physical health. It offers many benefits, like preventing diseases and helping with their treatment and recovery. When kids are active, they tend to stay that way as they grow up, which is good for their health in the long run.[2]

'Kaki, just like you make investments and savings for the future, a gym is also an investment for his future. It is like giving your child the lifelong gift of good health.'

'But, Manan . . .' she tried to argue.

I assured her, 'Gym workouts will not impact the epiphyseal growth plates (responsible for gaining height) adversely in any way as long as they are done with proper form and technique and under the supervision of a qualified fitness trainer. With proper guidance and supervision, Mohit can embark on his fitness journey safely. You don't have to worry!'

Trying to lighten the mood, I suggested, 'Why not turn it into a family affair? You and Kaka could join Mohit at the gym. It's a fantastic way to motivate each other and stay fit.'

There was a moment of silence on the other end before Mamta Kaki finally relented. 'Alright, Manan. Mohit can join the gym,' she conceded, her tone softer now.

Before ending the call, she added with a chuckle, 'And by the way, I've learnt a new recipe. I'll make it for you when you come over next.'

I couldn't help but smile at her gesture. 'I will come on a Monday when I am fasting. *Bilkul riks nahi lena re, baba*,' I teased in my best Baburao voice from the cult classic *Hera Pheri*.

We both laughed, the tension from earlier dissipating. Mohit's gymming journey was off to a promising start and the magic of science had worked yet again.

Sperm in the Hot Seat

Laptop Lore Debunked

One routine weekend, my wife and I were out running errands when I bumped into an old friend, Akhil. He was lugging around a large, unmarked box. Curiosity got the better of me and I asked, 'Hey, what's in the box?'

Akhil grinned and explained, 'Oh, this? I found someone online who makes these amazing laptop holders for cars. The best part is, it's detachable and foldable, so you can carry it with you even if you're travelling in a cab and still use it.'

Intrigued, I probed further, 'Why do you need a laptop holder for a car?'

He sighed, 'My workload has skyrocketed over the last few months and I spend a lot of time in cabs, trying to juggle commuting and working. My wife was worried about the exposure to laptops and its potential impact on my sperm count. We have been planning for a baby for some time now, you see!' He blushed and added, 'Then I came across this gadget, and it seemed like the perfect solution to my problem.'

I laughed, 'So this nifty gadget is saving your work-life balance and your future family all at once?'

Akhil chuckled. 'Exactly! It's a game-changer.'

I smiled and said, 'Sorry to break your heart, bro! But no notable connection has ever been observed between the use of laptops and the parameters of sperm quality,'[1]

Lifestyle factors play a major role in male infertility worldwide. Research indicates that sperm quality is primarily influenced by factors such as obesity, nicotine addiction and alcohol consumption.[2] Other secondary factors include air pollution, the use of pesticides and harmful chemicals and exposure to excessive heat.[3]

The most commonly ignored reasons are smoking and alcohol,[4] not to mention many underlying health issues like diabetes and stress, which can impact sperm count.[5]

I took a deep breath and paused for his reaction.

Akhil sighed, 'All morning, I have been contemplating opting for WFH for the next few months and moving to a desktop after hearing what my wife said. And now I learn this!'

I added, 'WFH is a good option. You will get to spend more time with her. The other things will automatically fall into place. You don't need to move to a desktop or anything, if you know what I mean.' And I winked.

The way Akhil's face turned red told me I had hit the bull's eye.

The Weight Loss Chronicles

Unveiling Apple Cider Vinegar's True Effects

WhatsApp groups are a mixed bag in today's world. You join them to avoid missing out, but they quickly become a pain point with their endless messages, ranging from morning greetings to deep discussions on various topics like politics, space exploration, health and relationships. And it doesn't stop there! Sometimes, late-night personal rants leave you puzzled about how to respond. Are they seeking advice, sympathy or just sharing? Should you react with a thumbs-up or a heart emoji? It's enough to make you wish for online etiquette classes.

Thanks to WhatsApp, today we all are a part of numerous groups, spanning from school and college to the workplace, cousins and other friends. Picture my astonishment as a doctor when I stumbled upon a message one morning from a group member boasting about their newfound ritual of guzzling apple cider vinegar each morning in their quest for weight loss and lower blood pressure.

I recognized the sender. We had once been friends, and witnessing him succumb to such internet gimmicks was disheartening. The pain inflicted by this message made my heart dance to its own version of 'Dard-e-disco' as it struggled to cope with the shock.

Typically, I avoid commenting on personal posts, often just reacting with emojis to happy news or updates. But this one . . . it felt urgent, like a cry for help. I wrestled with the dilemma all morning until during lunchtime, I finally broke my own rule of silence and responded to the message with some unsolicited advice.

'Apple Cider Vinegar does not help in weight loss':[1] I typed it and sent it to the group.

At this hour, when the group was typically buzzing with activity, it was strangely quiet. Seizing the opportunity, I decided to share everything that was on my mind with them.

Neither is it some magical potion for blood pressure,[2] nor is it a magic bullet for your metabolism.[3] Conversely, apple cider vinegar also comes with its own set of side effects. For starters, your body might struggle to handle the acidic overload, potentially causing acid reflux. ACV is potent enough to affect your tooth enamel. Over time, it could also impact your kidneys.[4]

Once, there was a study conducted to assess the effect of apple cider vinegar on weight loss.[5] Participants not only consumed apple cider vinegar but also reduced their calorie intake and hit the gym, presumably while waiting for the magic potion to work.

I had barely clicked send when the original poster countered, 'But I've witnessed remarkable outcomes within my own circles, in addition to the guidance provided by my nutritionist.'

'Just like other supplements, apple cider vinegar can't substitute for a healthy lifestyle. While it might offer some advantages for our bodies, we still require more research to fully grasp the health perks and drawbacks of apple cider vinegar.'

One member, genuinely worried, asked, 'What's your advice, then?'

'There's no evidence to back up most of these apple cider vinegar claims.[6] You are better off working out and leading a healthy lifestyle for your weight loss and other health issues rather than looking for some magic elixirs on the Internet. After all, you don't want any "Dard-e-disco" in your life! Do you?'

He quickly responded, 'Only disco. No *dard*, doctor!' The original poster sent a gif of a bare-chested Shah Rukh Khan standing with open arms in what appeared to be a still from the song 'Dard-e-disco'.

Interpreting the number of hearts on my recent post, I concluded that all was well in the end and that apple cider vinegar had found its rightful place—in the kitchen, as a food ingredient. And so I went back to my work.

Zero Fat, Maximum Fiction

The Deceptive Reality of 'Fat-Free' Labels

One weekend, I decided to host a potluck party with a few of my neighbours at our house. The harsh summer had just ended and we'd had our first rains, making it perfect weather for a get-together in the building's common area. As the evening progressed, it was delightful catching up with everyone as they arrived, each one bearing trays of food. One neighbour brought starters while another made nimbu pani and aam panna for all of us. Mrs Khan, my next-door neighbour, brought biryani, and Mr Sharma baked his favourite dark chocolate fudge for everyone.

We chatted and waited for Naman, the last resident on our floor, to arrive. He finally showed up with a bag full of what looked like store-bought snacks. Curious, I asked, 'What's in the bag?'

He replied, 'Fat-free crispies for us to munch on!'

Surprised, I asked him why fat-free, to which he responded, 'One of my colleagues had a heart attack a few months ago at work. He was asked to reduce his cholesterol levels and fat consumption. It scared us all, so we've switched to fat-free food both at work and at home for better health. What better way to introduce my neighbours to this little-known gem?' he quipped.

I nodded, because it made sense that they were now more mindful of their dietary choices.

As I took a bite of the snack, I couldn't help but interject, 'You know, not all foods labelled as "fat-free" are actually free of fat because sometimes food labels can be misleading. Even if a product is labelled as "fat-free", it might still contain small amounts of fat.'

Nowadays, supermarket aisles are brimming with fat-free products, ranging from snacks, chips and cookies to bread and juices. However, if your goal is to adopt a low-fat diet to manage cholesterol levels, relying on fat-free options isn't a silver bullet.[1]

We often assume that products labelled as fat-free are healthier choices compared to their full-fat counterparts. But that's not necessarily true. Consider this: when fat is removed from a product, much of its taste is lost as well. To make up for this, food manufacturers often add other ingredients[2] like sugar, flour, thickeners and salt. These ingredients restore the flavour while increasing the calorie content. So, while that 'low-fat' snack in your cart may have less fat than the regular one, it likely contains more additives and calories, making it not much better for you.[3]

Naman looked at me questioningly, so I explained.

'Bro, please don't stress about it. It can still be done. Instead of solely focusing on whether a product is fat-free or not, it's important to look at the overall nutritional value. So I suggest you opt for snacks that are high in fibres, vitamins and minerals, and low on added sugars and unhealthy fats.[4] Leave out any fried snacks or ones with large amounts of preservatives.'

I could sense the air becoming tense. So I tried to lighten the mood. 'Just ring me up whenever you need a healthy food detective to track down those elusive, better-for-you snacks. *Main Hoon Naa*, Naman!' I mimicked Shah Rukh Khan.

Follicle Follies

Debunking the Biotin Hair Fall Hoax!

One weekend, we visited my aunt, Meenal Masi, in Ahmedabad. The plan for the day was to go sightseeing.

My cousin shouted, 'Coming in 5! Will just take a quick shower and we can leave.'

'Okay,' I told her and made myself a cup of coffee.

Holidays are meant to relax. So I took my cuppa and started reading the newspaper lying nearby while sitting on the swing in their balcony. The cool and gentle breeze added magic to the lazy morning.

Fifteen minutes later, I had finished my coffee but there was no sign of my cousin. I waited patiently while strolling around the balcony for a while more. Soon, I heard her footsteps.

'Hey, sorry I'm late,' Alisha apologized, drying her hair with a towel.

'No worries. Everything okay?' I asked, concerned by her dishevelled appearance.

Alisha let out a sigh, running a hand through her hair. 'Not really. I've been dealing with a lot of hair fall lately and I just don't know what to do about it.'

I frowned sympathetically, knowing how distressing hair fall can be.

Alisha nodded, her expression hopeful. 'Yeah, I've been taking biotin supplements, thinking they would help strengthen my hair and prevent it from falling out. But so far, I haven't seen any improvement.'

I raised an eyebrow, intrigued by her choice of remedy. 'Biotin supplements? Is your friend a dermatologist?'

Alisha nodded, frustration evident in her voice. 'No . . . ooo! I thought they would be a quick fix, but it seems like they're not doing much for me.'

Just then, Meenal Masi joined us. 'What is being discussed so seriously?' she asked.

Alisha wasted no time in venting her frustrations. 'We're talking about hair fall, and how I've been taking biotin supplements to try and stop it. But it doesn't seem to be working.'

Meenal Masi raised an eyebrow, looking thoughtful. 'Hmm, you never listen to me. I told you to stop using all those shampoos and use shikakai like me. I've heard mixed reviews about biotin supplements. Some people say they work wonders, while others claim they're just a waste of money.'

Alisha nodded in agreement, looking increasingly exasperated. 'At this rate, I am afraid I will go bald soon.'

I leaned back in my chair, contemplating the situation. 'Do you know there is insufficient evidence to support biotin working as a supplement for good hair?'[1]

'WHAT?' Alisha and Meenal Masi almost let out a scream.

'Please relax!' I said and explained.

Biotin is a water-soluble vitamin that acts as a crucial helper in various metabolic processes. Its affordability and easy availability have made it a popular choice for consumers seeking to improve their health and the appearance of their hair and nails. But there is no scientific evidence to back its claim of working magic on hair and nails.[2]

'What about my hair now?' Alisha was on the verge of tears.

'Hair fall can occur due to various reasons, ranging from stress and side effects of medications to underlying illnesses like thyroid or iron deficiency. It is important to find the root cause of the hair fall to find the right solution.'[3]

Alisha and Meenal Masi stared at me as I said, 'At this moment, you're essentially taking a shot in the dark.'

Both were silent for a while before they spoke together, 'Maybe we should see a dermatologist!'

That one word was like pure magic to my ears as I felt relieved that they had finally understood the situation better.

'Ma, I will come back in the evening and make an appointment with the dermatologist for this week,' she told Meenal Masi while picking up her purse.

'Take one for me too . . .' Meenal Masi sheepishly added just as we were about to leave.

Alisha and I both facepalmed together.

Sweat Equity

How Much Fat Are You Really Burning?

L ast week, I hit the gym in the evening as usual and came back home, only to bump into Mohsin, one of the residents of the colony, in the parking lot.

Mohsin was in his early thirties and had a clearly visible paunch. His body type was heavy. Of late, he had taken to working out, including stretching and walking, in the common garden. Mohsin was dressed in Nike gear from head to toe and was sweating profusely. He came straight to me, his expression a mix of curiosity and frustration.

'Hey Manan, how are you?' he said, his tone friendly yet perplexed.

'I am well, Mohsin. How are you?'

That's when he noticed my gym bag and asked, 'Back from the gym?' I nodded.

'I also work out here,' he said pointing at the common garden.

After a brief pause, he probed, 'I wanted to ask you something. You spend so much money at the air-conditioned gym, which doesn't even make you sweat.

They say the more you sweat, the more fat you burn. Why don't you also start working out here in the open?'

'It's a common misconception that sweating profusely equates to fat loss,[1] but the truth is far from it,' I told him.

Scientifically, there's no direct connection[2] between the two. Sweating is simply your body's way of cooling down when your internal temperature rises during exercise. It's not an indicator of how many calories or how much fat you're burning.[3]

His eyebrows shot up in surprise, clearly intrigued by this revelation. 'Really? But then why do I sweat so much during my workouts if it's not helping me lose weight?'

I leaned in, ready to drop some knowledge bombs. 'Well, think of sweating as your body's built-in air conditioning system. When you exercise, your muscles generate heat, causing your body temperature to rise. In response, your sweat glands kick into high gear to release moisture on to your skin, which then evaporates and cools you down. It's all about regulating your body temperature, not shedding the kilos.[4]

'Let me guess—you are wondering that if sweat does not lead to weight loss, then what does? Am I right?' I asked him, looking at his perplexed face.

He nodded with a smile.

'It all boils down to creating a calorie deficit.[5] That means burning more calories[6] than you consume through a combination of exercise and a balanced diet. Focus on challenging workouts, consistency and making healthier food choices, and you'll see results.'[7]

He seemed relieved to finally have some clarity on the matter. 'Whoa! Science and maths coming together to create magic. I guess I need to be patient for the magic to happen.'

I clapped him on the back, 'Yes, and remember Nike's slogan—Just Do It! That should be your approach to working out!'

I don't know what it is about Nike, but it brought a huge smile to his face.

Sweet Debate

Are Jaggery and Honey Sugar-Coated Lies?

A doctor's daily routine is a roller coaster ride filled with surprises, challenges and a wide range of emotions. Each day brings new faces, new stories and new opportunities to make a positive impact on someone's life. Doctors are constantly reminded of the complex tapestry of human experiences, from listening to funny anecdotes to witnessing moments of deep trauma and pain.

And then there are those days when we doctors stumble upon some new, 'interesting' information. Like the day I discovered the myth that honey was a healthier alternative to sugar. And no, it wasn't from a WhatsApp joke, believe it or not. It was an actual patient who had sworn by this and came to see me. What happened next is anyone's guess, like the plot twists in a Bollywood movie!

My day started like any other routine day at the clinic. Patients coming in and out, sharing their health concerns and seeking advice. However, one particular patient caught my attention—Mr Sharma, a regular visitor for his routine check-ups.

'Good morning, Mr Sharma! How have you been?' I greeted him warmly as he settled into the chair across my desk.

'I'm doing okay, doctor. But I've been having some knee pain lately,' Mr Sharma replied, rubbing his knee with a grimace.

'Let me take a look at your reports,' I said, reaching for his file. As I glanced through his recent test results, something caught my eye—his blood sugar levels were higher than usual.

'Mr Sharma, have you made any changes to your diet recently?' I inquired, raising an eyebrow.

'Oh, yes, doctor! I've completely cut out sugar from my diet. No more sweets or desserts for me,' he exclaimed proudly.

I nodded, but a nagging suspicion crept into my mind. Something didn't quite add up. 'Can you tell me more about your diet? What do you usually eat in a day?'

Mr Sharma proceeded to describe his daily meals in detail, and that's when it hit me—jaggery and honey! He was consuming them in copious amounts, believing them to be healthy alternatives to sugar.

'Mr Sharma, I hate to break it to you, but jaggery and honey are also forms of sugar,' I explained gently. 'They may be natural, but they still raise your blood sugar levels and can contribute to health problems if consumed excessively.'

Mr Sharma's eyes widened in surprise. 'But I thought they were safe! I've been told that jaggery and honey are better than refined sugar.'

I chuckled softly. 'It's a common misconception, Mr Sharma. While jaggery and honey do have some nutritional benefits, they're still high in calories and can spike your blood sugar levels if consumed in large quantities.'

Jaggery, like sugar, is also made from sugarcane.[1] It is a concentrated product of cane juice without separation of the molasses[2] and crystals. It contains up to 50 per cent sucrose, up to 20 per cent invert sugars and some other insoluble matter such as ash, proteins and bagasse fibres.[3] A high-calorie sweetener, jaggery contains minerals, proteins, glucose and fructose, making it a healthier option compared to white sugar when consumed in moderation.[4] However, a study found that the sugar levels after consuming jaggery were identical to the sugar levels after consuming white sugar, making it an unsafe option for diabetics.[5]

On the other hand, honey has a lower glycemic index compared to sugar and jaggery. However, diabetes patients still face obstacles and challenges when using honey.[6]

Seeing the concern on Mr Sharma's face, I reassured him. 'But don't worry! Now that we know the culprit, we can make some adjustments to your diet and get your blood sugar levels back on track. It's all about finding the right balance.'

Together, we discussed healthier alternatives and came up with a plan that included going completely sugar-free, this time without jaggery and honey as well.

Turmeric

Fairy Dust or Just a Spicy Hoax?

O ur home often welcomes visiting relatives, and on one occasion, a distant relative stayed with us. It was customary for guests to bring gifts ranging from sweets and clothes to books. However, this time, our guest surprised us with something unexpected: a packet of turmeric pills.

Intrigued by the unusual gift, we exchanged puzzled glances. Sensing our confusion, our relative enthusiastically explained, 'You know I had gone to visit my guru in the Himalayas. I got these turmeric pills from there as they have the purest quality.'

I smiled, not knowing what to say as she continued, 'These pills have this compound called curcumin, which is amazing for fighting inflammation and boosting antioxidants. It is a popular choice for combating diseases like cancer, infections and inflammatory conditions.'

She added further, 'I have been living with rheumatoid arthritis for years now. On Guruji's advice, I started taking these pills early this year and have seen great results in my pain. With this,' she handed the packet of turmeric pills to my wife and said, 'I wish you all good health. You should eat these pills twice a day to stay healthy.'

Just as we were about to call it a night, she insisted on hot milk with turmeric for all of us, claiming it was beneficial for our health. That's when I realized it was time to dispel this myth once and for all.

'Kaki, turmeric is good only in small quantities. Too much turmeric can be harmful.' I tried to reason with her.

'E . . . na . . . na . . . have. Back at our place, we even give it to pregnant women and newborn babies. It is very good for health and has zero side effects,' she argued.

'Kaki, that is exactly where you are wrong,' I sat next to her and continued,' According to a study by WHO, there is no clinical data[1] to establish the safety of this product during pregnancy, lactation and in children.'

For centuries, certain countries have incorporated curcumin into their diets at doses of less than 100mg/day.[2] It is harmless for short-term usage at doses of up to 8 gm/day.[3] However, the long-term safety of turmeric as a compounded medicine remains unclear[4] due to various factors. Diarrhoea[5] is the most common side effect. It just doesn't end here. It has also been observed to contribute to oxidative stress in cases of acute vitiligo,[6] not to mention its antiplatelet effects.[7] High-absorption formulations found in turmeric are toxic to the liver.[8]

'And to talk about curcumin treatment for maintaining remission of rheumatoid arthritis,[9] well, it's just as effective as no treatment at all!' I concluded, half expecting her to understand.

Kaki sat quietly with a grim look on her face.

So I tried to end the discussion by saying, 'Turmeric belongs in the kitchen. Its role is to add taste to our food and not be a medicine.' Still no response from her.

'Please get rid of these pills, Kaki,' I requested. 'I will schedule an appointment for you with me at the clinic while you are here. Let's look for a proper solution backed by science instead of these quick fixes that can cause more harm than healing.'

To this, she finally looked at me and nodded.

Hyaluronic Acid

The Hype and the Hilarity!

It's **Ananya's birthday,'** the notification from Google Calendar said on my phone.

As I dialled her number to wish her a happy birthday, I could barely contain my excitement. My childhood friend, Ananya, was turning thirty today.

'Hey, happy birthday!' I wished her.

'Thank you!' Ananya's excitement was palpable in her voice. She was over the moon about her special day and I couldn't wait to hear her plans.

'So how does it feel to be thirty?' I asked cheerfully.

'You know, it feels great, but you won't believe what my parents got me for my birthday. It's incredible!' she exclaimed.

'Oh, do tell me! What's this amazing gift?' I inquired, genuinely intrigued.

'My parents got me this entire skincare package at my favourite skin clinic! It includes hyaluronic acid injections and other skincare services, and it's going to last for a whole year. Isn't that just fantastic?' she gushed.

As she raved about her gift, I couldn't help but feel a little concerned.

'Ananya, that's great and all, but are you sure about this? Hyaluronic acid injections can have side effects, and they're not necessarily something everyone needs, especially at your age,' I said cautiously.

'Oh, come on, Manan! Don't be such a killjoy. I've read so much about it, and everyone says women over thirty should start getting these treatments. My parents thought it would be the perfect gift and I trust them,' she replied confidently.

For a few seconds, I debated if I should argue with her on her birthday or leave it for another day. I finally gave in.

'Ananya, while hyaluronic acid treatments can be beneficial, they also come with their fair share of side effects.'

Did You Know?

Being informed about evidence-based treatment is crucial but can be challenging, because of which many people often resort to anti-ageing cosmetics that lack rigorous scientific backing.[1]

'Like what?' Ananya was irritated now.

'Oh, there are so many! Who knows, you might even end up having an interesting allergic reaction[2] to a particular brand or formulation.'

'Huh? I was told there are no side effects.' The surprise in her tone betrayed the fact that my words had had some impact on her.

'Moreover, hyaluronic acid is not recommended for people with bleeding conditions, those who are pregnant, those who have sensitive skin and those who are prone to anaphylactic reactions to various bacteria.'[3]

Research has uncovered acute, short-term or chronic toxicity[4] in people who use hyaluronic acid. Most importantly, the effects of hyaluronic acid are not permanent.[5] It is a cycle[6] where you do it once and have to keep repeating it to ensure the effects stay.

For any skin-related issues, always consult a dermatologist and only follow treatments and procedures recommended or approved by them for your specific skin needs. Don't just randomly opt for cosmetic treatments without expert assessment and advice.

'Oh God, what *is* permanent in today's times?' Ananya lamented.

'Well, there are a few permanent and even risk-free ways to take care of your skin. Like drinking enough water, getting at least 8 hours of sleep, eating a nutritious diet, working out and leading a healthy and active lifestyle. Also, meeting friends regularly to have a good laugh about stupid jokes!'

Ananya started laughing at this and soon, I joined in.

'So, when are we meeting?' I asked.

'Soon, I promise. But before that, I need to find some way to encash this voucher at the skin clinic without causing any severe damage. Gotta go now, will talk to you later!' The call was disconnected and I was happy that the day had been saved with science and humour intact.

Bright Ideas

The Screen Time Saga

It was a long weekend because a local festival fell on Monday, so a bunch of us friends decided to head to a friend's farmhouse in Alibaug with our spouses and children. The plan was to relax and enjoy some quality time together. The farmhouse was well-stocked and had plenty of staff and caretakers, so we had little to worry about.

We arrived on Saturday morning and spent the rest of the day indoors. In the evening, we went to the beach and had a great time playing in the waves with the children. After a long day and enjoying a hearty meal of farm-fresh wood-fired pizzas made by the farmhouse cook, we decided to call it a night.

As I walked to our room, I heard my friend Amar's voice: 'No means no!' He was loudly saying this to his five-year-old, who was engrossed in a game on the iPad.

The house lights had been dimmed and Amar was concerned about his son's eyes being exposed to the screen in the dark. 'You'll damage your eyes, *bachcha*! Then you'll need thick glasses. You don't want that, do you? Now be a good boy and give the iPad to Papa.

'Nooooo! Papa, just 10 more minutes. I am about to win this round!' His son was in no mood to listen.

I approached Amar and offered, 'Bro, if you want to get some rest, I can stay with him for a while and make sure he falls asleep soon. Don't worry!'

'That's not the issue, Manan,' Amar replied. 'I'm concerned about his eyes being exposed to the screen in the dark. I don't want him to harm his eyes like this. If he really wants to play, he can come inside the room and play. At least the lights are on there.'

'Bro, you know that's not true,' I insisted, but the blank expression on Amar's face told me he was taken aback.

With the spirits of science by my side, I rattled off:

'Amar, watching TV or any screen in the dark has no adverse effect[1] on our eyes.' As soon as I uttered those words, I witnessed the child's expression light up with joy. He pumped his fist in the air and exclaimed, 'Yes!' before eagerly returning to his game.

Seeing Amar still puzzled, I clarified, 'External lighting doesn't affect eye strain; it's the brightness of the screen that is harmful.[2] Prolonged exposure to any type of screen can dry the eyes and cause eye strain or eye fatigue.'[3]

While there is no specific number of hours that can be considered prolonged exposure for children and adolescents, the Indian Academy of Paediatrics[4] says, 'It is important to balance screen time with other activities that are required for overall development.'

It's recommended to keep your screen at least 20 cm away from your eyes and take regular breaks.

Saying this, I glanced at the child engrossed in his game. 'Hold on a sec!' I signalled, then swiftly took the iPad from him, adjusted the screen brightness and handed it back.

Tip: The optimal screen brightness[5] for eye protection is one that adjusts to ambient light. It should be bright enough to read text without squinting or straining, but not so bright that it bathes your face in artificial light. To find this balance, hold a sheet of paper next to your screen and adjust the display to match the paper's brightness. In a well-lit room, the paper—and consequently, the screen—will need to be brighter.

Amar's expression eased as he watched, and he smiled at me. 'I'm taking your advice, Manan and letting this little champ play for now!' he said, tousling his child's hair affectionately.

'Yes, please! The only precautionary measure that is recommended to prevent any damage to the eye is keeping the eyes moist.'[6]

We had taken just a few steps towards our room when the lively voice from the phone declared the end of the game, proclaiming our champ as the winner—much like science had triumphed that night.

Tipsy Truths

Unveiling Moderation and Myths

Let's play a game of 'never have I ever'. Answer yes to all the things from the list below that you have never done before.

Never Have I Ever

- Drunk too much alcohol.
- Had more than a few drinks.
- Made drinking daily a habit.

If you nodded yes to all of this, congratulations, you are a social drinker!

But wait, there's a while to the toast! The ultimate truth is there's no such thing as a social drinker—you're either a drinker or you are not. By using the tag 'social drinker', you are fooling absolutely no one except yourself.

Alcohol in any form or quantity is not safe for our body.[1] Sipping in moderation isn't quite the strategic manoeuvre it's cracked up to be!

Just like those annoying Instagram dance reels on trending songs, alcohol seems to have a way of making almost every part of our body cringe a little. And we are just getting started.

Alcohol affects our brain and nerves in different ways, such as slowing down the brain, harming brain cells, tightening brain tissues and reducing nerve activity, leading to potential injury.[2] Consumption of alcohol has an adverse impact on the cardiovascular system.[3] From causing early menopause[4] to cancer,[5] the spirits linger everywhere. Alcohol can cause serious damage to the pancreas,[6] the liver,[7] the gut,[8] the limbs[9]. . . Ah, the list of mischief goes on forever. And the damage? Well, let's just say it has its own season pass!

And what's the grand prize for your moderate sipping marathon? Absolutely nothing!

And no, there are no safety nets here. There is no safe level[10] of alcohol consumption, as per medical science.

Contrarily, saying no to alcohol comes with an epic line-up of benefits in that arena.

First, you become the designated driver extraordinaire for every social shindig and office bash. And as a bonus, you get the golden chance to dazzle everyone with your astonishing anomaly: 'You're not a drinker? Why ever not?'

I know, I know, that lone mug of beer or solitary glass of champagne is tempting at a party, a gathering or a bad day at work. These temptations are mischievous troublemakers in disguise. They tiptoe into our systems and disrupt it slowly, away from prying eyes.

So next time you raise that glass, remember: behind the fizz and froth lies Pandora's box of surprises!

Need more reasons?

The Great Sugar Conspiracy

Separating Fact from Fiction

One evening, after the chaos of a busy workday, I found myself rushing home, eager to hit the gym for some much-needed stress relief. Just as I was mentally gearing up for a workout, I bumped into my friendly neighbours—a delightful couple with an even more delightful five-year-old. Engaging in conversation, the husband kindly extended an invitation to their child's upcoming birthday party, which was the weekend after at 7 p.m. However, before he could finish, his wife interjected with a firm 'No, 6 o'clock sharp!' They started whispering among themselves.

Sensing a minor disagreement, I turned to the husband, expecting him to clarify.

With a sheepish grin, he admitted, 'We're still finalizing the details.'

I couldn't help but ask, 'Is there some confusion?'

'Ah, yes!' the husband replied. 'And who better than you to help us, Doc.'

The husband explained, 'My wife believes that feeding cake to kids later in the evening will cause them to be high on sugar. They'll stay hyperactive and that will disrupt their sleep schedule, causing a lot of problems for us parents.'

'And how do you know this?' I was getting inquisitive now.

'Well . . . WhatsApp,' the wife confessed.

'Oh, come on now, it's 2024. You cannot believe everything you see on WhatsApp!' I exclaimed, shaking my head dramatically.

'There is no evidence that sugar makes kids hyperactive,'[1] I added, after a long pause.

Their faces resembled blank canvases, each sporting a sizeable question mark as they gazed back at me in utter bewilderment. The wife seemed momentarily speechless, her expression a blend of surprise and confusion. I gave a subtle nod, silently urging them to react before I proceeded.

'Now imagine a bustling birthday bash with kids running around, giggles echoing and excitement in the air. Whether they've had loads of cake or not, the party atmosphere alone is enough to fuel their exuberance. The setting also has a huge role to play when children become hyperactive.[2] Sugar alone cannot and should not be blamed.'

The wife opened her mouth to ask something when I interrupted her.

'I know what you are about to say and no! It is still not the sugar. I still stand by my statement. There is no connection between sugar and hyperactive[3] children, even without a birthday party. When you offer chocolate to a kid as a reward for good behaviour or great results, the excitement of having achieved something is high enough for them to become hyperactive.[4]

'And before you blame me, I want to clarify. I'm not here to defend sugar or call it healthy. It's bad news for both kids and adults, wreaking all sorts of havoc on everything from our teeth to our kidneys. But let's not go pinning every problem on it, shall we?'

The husband sighed in relief and looked at his wife: 'See, I have been telling you. A little sugar will not turn our child into a mini-Shinchan!'

The wife, her eyes wide with realization, nodded eagerly. 'Wow, Doc! You've just given me a whole new perspective. Thank you for inspiring me to be kinder to my child!'

I smiled, 'Let kids be kids and have fun. If you're seeking inspiration, channel your inner Amrish Puri from the climax of *DDLJ*, not the one before that. Loosen the grip on your child's hand and whisper, "*Jaa, je lee apni zindagi* (Go, live your life)!"'

As I uttered those words, they burst into unexpected laughter, almost resembling hyperactive children, and yes, it was due to my joke, not a sugar high.

Straightening Out the Lies

Chiropractic Myths Exposed

'Hey Hetvi, guess what? We're gearing up for a wild weekend getaway to Goa! Just us cousins, reuniting for some epic adventures. Wanna join?' I eagerly messaged my cousin.

'Ah, wish I could, but I've got to play chauffeur for Dad's chiropractor appointment,' Hetvi replied, dropping the 'C' word like a bomb. Instantly, my fingers flew across the screen to dial her number.

'Please tell me you're kidding,' I blurted out the moment she picked up.

'Kidding about what?' came her puzzled response.

'The chiropractor visit? You're pulling my leg, right?' I pressed, hoping for a different answer.

'Why would I joke about that?' Hetvi shot back.

'Because you don't want to come with us?' I countered, a note of desperation creeping into my voice.

'Believe me, I wish I was! Dad's been on a health roller coaster lately. We've done the whole doctor–hospital–blood report routine, but no luck. Then, out of the blue, Raju

Uncle suggested this chiropractor miracle worker. After weeks of waiting, we've finally snagged an appointment this weekend. So I'm on duty.' She let out a sigh of exasperation.

'Can I tag along? I have always wanted to see a Munnabhai in real life!' I insisted.

'Huh?' She sounded befuddled.

'Well, chiropractors are not doctors. You see, like that character Munnabhai, played by Sanjay Dutt?'

'This is serious, Manan.' Her agitation was evident in her voice now.

'And I am serious too,' I clarified and continued, 'Chiropractic is a form of alternative medicine without any scientific backing. Medically, there is no proof that it works and helps people heal. On the contrary, we have more cases of people being grievously injured or worse, losing their lives due to this.'[1]

I could hear her pacing back and forth, her nervousness evident in her heavy breathing over the phone as she processed everything I had shared, grappling with its implications. She was too shocked to respond, so I kept going.

'Chiropractic is not a recommended solution for any spinal complaints.[2] I know chiropractors suggest that issues with joints, particularly the spine, impact overall health and that spinal adjustments enhance well-being. But that's not true!'[3]

Solid evidence indicates that chiropractic is no more effective than other treatments in alleviating pain and enhancing function in individuals with long-standing lower back pain.[4] Even more concerning, it can result in immediate fatality in certain instances.[5] In 2016, a model named Katie May[6] died because her chiropractor ruptured an artery in her neck.

'It worked wonders for Raju Uncle's wife . . .' Hetvi argued.

'There are success stories, but only short-term. Chiropractic care doesn't provide lasting relief from pain,'[7] I tried to explain.

'Manan, you are confusing me with this medical gibberish now!' She was losing her calm, I could sense.

'Okay, how about this? Mutual fund investments are subject to market risk. Please read the offer documents carefully,' I said in one breath without a pause.

'I just heard the words 'risk' and 'carefully'. Say that again.'

'That's all that was needed, Hetvi.'

For a moment, all that filled the call was the gentle hum of the fan in the background, accompanied by the distant murmur of evening traffic growing outside my home.

I heard her exhale heavily before saying, 'I'm torn between relief that I shielded my father from a potentially risky medical intervention and disappointment that we're still at a loss for a solution to his ongoing pain.'

'Let me come over this weekend to see him. I will also check his medical reports and start his treatment,' I suggested.

'Sure, that would be perfect. Thank you, Manan.' But Hetvi was still obviously concerned.

'*Bole toh*, tension *nahi lene ka*, Mamu!' I mimicked Munnabhai (Mumbai slang that translates to don't worry).'

Hetvi giggled, proving once again that the only prescription from Munnabhai that truly works is laughter.

The Java Jive

A Tale of Black Coffee and Productivity

As a dedicated friend and occasional sidekick in my cousin Kartik's weekend escapade projects, I found myself knee-deep in conversations, caffeine and camaraderie. Each Saturday and Sunday, his home office turned into a hub of creativity and chaos, fuelled by endless cups of black coffee and even more banter.

One rainy afternoon, amid endless to-do lists and frustrating follow-ups, I got up to refill my java. Humming a song, I went to heat up some water and make a cup of black coffee when my cousin passed an acerbic commented.

'Oh gosh, Manan,' Kartik exclaimed, shaking his head in mock disbelief, 'the number of black coffees you have in a day is giving me a headache! How are you still standing after all that java floating in you? Looks like if someone were to cut you open, black coffee would flow out instead of blood!'

I couldn't help but chuckle at his dramatic declaration. 'Bro, tell me you are jealous of my productivity without telling me you are jealous!'

'Jealous of you?' Kartik was surprised.

'Yes, because my productivity is higher than yours! *Jalta hai tu* Majnu!' I said, mimicking Nana Patekar from *Welcome*.

Kartik started laughing loudly at this and I joined him soon. As we high-fived on this, I broke the real news to him.

'To tell you about the magic called coffee, I will have to take you back in time, my friend,' I started with dramatic flair.

'The effects of coffee on human health and disease have been acknowledged for centuries. As early as the late sixteenth century, it was noted that coffee sped up digestion and elevated heart rate.'[1]

Black coffee is not just a drink—it's a lifeline, a source of energy and a fountain of productivity all rolled into one steaming cup. A plain black cup of coffee has so few calories,[2] it's practically on a diet of its own!

Not only does it provide a much-needed caffeine boost to kickstart the day, but it also enhances focus, sharpens cognitive function and boosts overall mental alertness.[3] Coffee drinking is strongly linked to better liver health, showing significant and consistent benefits for conditions like fibrosis, cirrhosis, chronic liver disease and liver cancer.[4]

Kartik raised an eyebrow in curiosity, his interest piqued by my passionate monologue on the virtues of our favourite dark elixir.

'But wait, there's more!' I continued, unable to contain my enthusiasm. 'Did you know that black coffee is also an excellent pre-workout beverage? Its caffeine content acts as a natural stimulant, increasing adrenaline levels and improving physical performance during exercise. Plus, it helps to mobilize fat stores and enhance metabolism too!'[5]

It is important to remember that black coffee is best (no milk, no sugar) and only up to 400 mg[6] a day (to know more about coffee chronicles, turn to page 237).

'Oh gosh . . . all this coffee talk is making me crave it now!' Kartik screamed.

'Welcome to the dark side, bro!' I winked at him. 'And wait till you taste the coffee I make for you.'

Second-Hand Smoke

Blowing Away the Cloud of Misconception

I t was a typical weekend rendezvous with friends at our favourite restaurant. The ambience was lively, the aroma of food tantalizing and laughter filled the air as we settled into our cosy corner near the window.

As we exchanged stories and caught up on each other's lives, I couldn't help but notice a cloud of smoke drifting in from outside. 'Ugh, someone's smoking again,' I muttered, wrinkling my nose in distaste.

To my surprise, Shazad, one of my friends, chimed in, 'Last I checked, it's a free country and smoking isn't illegal here. Everyone's free to puff away to their heart's content, wherever and whenever they please. What's your problem, bro?'

'Passive smoking can be harmful to our health!' I shared.

'Oh, passive smoking isn't that harmful, Manan. You're worrying too much.' Shazad did not seem to be convinced.

I couldn't let that slide. With a knowing smile, I shared a deep dark secret.

'Well, now I know where your GPS gets all the wrong ideas from! Your stories of getting lost on the way to something important are iconic, bro.'

Did you know that passive smoking can actually be more harmful than smoking itself?

'Passive smoking, also known as second-hand smoking, is no laughing matter,' I continued, leaning in to emphasize my point. 'When you inhale second-hand smoke, you're exposed to over 4000 chemicals, out of which at least 250 chemicals[1] are known to be toxic or carcinogenic.'

Shazad's eyes widened in surprise and I knew I had his attention.

Passive smoking increases the risk of heart disease and respiratory conditions like asthma and bronchitis.[2] And it's especially dangerous for children and pregnant women. Research shows that both passive smoking and active smoking may similarly raise the likelihood of certain diseases, including female breast cancer,[3] allergic rhinitis, allergic dermatitis and food allergies.[4] Being exposed to environmental tobacco smoke may heighten the risk of developing lung cancer and cervical cancer.

'The list of illnesses caused by passive smoking is as endless as a never-ending horror story, getting scarier with every dramatic pause.' I paused to let my words sink in.

'No wonder I feel so terrible in that smoking area of my office. Must be my allergies!' Priya confessed.

Shazad seemed to be lost in thought for a while before he said, 'Cigarette smoking is so terrible, man! It just doesn't kill you, it also kills the person around you who inhales the smoke. All this for a few moments of cheap thrill, and at what cost?'

For a moment, we all exchanged glances and like clockwork, raised our hands to bow to Baba Shazad, who seemed to have finally found his awakening!

Fruity Gossip

Why It Is Best to Keep It Whole

Picture this: It's February and the wedding marathon is going strong! You're waltzing into your 3825th wedding in just two months. Your stomach has declared a hunger strike in every dialect known to man, so you've taken a solemn vow of abstinence from all things edible. However, Mr Mehta, whose daughter is the bride of the hour, is playing the persistent host and insists that you partake in something, anything, even if it's just a refreshing glass of freshly squeezed fruit juice at the wedding feast.

Just a few hours back, that was me—caught in the clutches of the relentless Mr Mehta! No amount of sweet talk could sway him from his mission. So I mustered up the courage to make a daring request.

'How about a plate of freshly cut fruits instead of those tempting juices?'

Mr Mehta graciously obliged. But, oh boy, the expressions on the onlookers' faces were priceless!

One of them couldn't resist and popped the million-dollar question, 'Manan, why on earth did you refuse those delightful juices?'

'Fruit juices are off my list for various reasons. Care to join me for a quick biology lesson?'

I now had the attention of others in the group. 'Yes, yes. Please enlighten us.'

'Let me share a story with you. Once, there was a man who decided to sustain himself solely on juices for six weeks. However, by the end of this period, he was diagnosed with acute renal failure. Any guesses as to why?'

Seeing their expressions, I pressed on without hesitation.

'This happened due to high oxalate levels. Oxalate is a substance found in some fruits, vegetables and nuts that can harm the kidneys.[1] Consuming fruit juice poses problems due to its high sugar content and insufficient fibre levels. Even if it's entirely natural, fruit juice packs a considerable amount of sugar and calories. Additionally, research suggests that consuming sucrose without its natural fibre, as is often the case with fruit juice, can lead to metabolic syndrome, liver damage and weight gain.'[2]

'I am on a liquid diet to lose weight and these juices never make me feel full,' Mr Solanki voiced his concern, prompting a collective sigh from the group.

'Juices never do that. Not the ones made at home. Not the preservative-free ones available in the market. Or the packaged ones sold in food bazaars. The fibre in whole fruit moderates the insulin response and enhances satiety,'[3] I added, chomping on an apple slice from my fruit plate.

The most senior member of the group, Mr Banerjee, finally spoke. 'Doctors always emphasize the importance of fruit consumption, but we often resort to juices for their convenience and availability. So, Manan, what do you advise?'

'Munch on those fruits until your teeth throw in the towel! Your body's counting on it, you know,' I quickly said.

'Wow, what a lifesaver! You've spared us from unhealthy choices,' Mr Solanki quipped, only to have Mr Banerjee add, 'And don't forget the money we've saved on the consultation fee! It's a win–win!'

Their laughter filled the room, each chuckle carrying the weight of newfound wisdom as they reached for more plates of whole fruits, leaving the glasses full of juice untouched.

Sunlight

Friend or Foe?

A few weeks ago, I arrived at my cousin's house at 9.30 a.m. to pick her up for a shopping expedition we had planned earlier. The exhibition, set up in open ground, featured a vibrant array of stalls full of handmade items ranging from home decor to handloom sarees and jewellery.

I was late and as soon as I stepped out of the car, I could see my cousin, Riya, waiting at her doorstep hesitantly.

'Hey Riya, ready to go?' I asked cheerfully.

Riya hesitated before responding, 'Actually, Manan, I was thinking . . . maybe we should wait until evening to go out.'

Surprised, I questioned, 'Why wait until evening? We've been planning this for days. I know I am a bit late due to traffic but we still have enough time to beat the evening rush.'

Riya looked down at her feet before replying, 'Well, you know how I am about sunlight. I've been reading a lot about how harmful it can be for the skin, and I just don't want to risk it.'

I couldn't help but chuckle at her concern. 'Scientists have acknowledged that exposure to sunlight's ultraviolet radiation (UVR) has negative[1] effects on human health. But on the other hand, it also has positive effects.'

The most well-known perk of sunlight is its power to boost your vitamin D levels; most vitamin D deficiencies stem from not getting enough time outdoors. And the best way to deal with the negative effects of UVR is using good sunscreen[2] (to know more about the uses of sunscreen, refer to page 6).

'But what about excessive UV rays causing skin damage?' Riya countered, looking genuinely worried.

I sighed, realizing that Riya's belief in the harmful effects of sunlight was deeply ingrained. 'Look, Riya, I understand your concern. But determining what qualifies as excessive exposure to UVR isn't a straightforward matter. Excessive essentially means exposure that is unreasonably high for your skin type given the level of UVR in the environment.'[3]

Avoiding exposure during the peak UV hours, typically between 10 a.m. and 3 p.m., is not practical for most people and is therefore not advisable. On the other hand, avoiding prolonged sun exposure could lead to more unwanted skin problems.[4]

Getting enough vitamin D through sunlight, diet or supplements can benefit your health. Low levels of vitamin D are linked to a higher risk of various health risks like type 2 diabetes, infections, cancer, multiple sclerosis and problems with thinking.[5]

'Ma, Manan is here. We are leaving!' She raised her voice to speak to her mother inside the house.

'Phew!' I wiped imaginary sweat beads from my forehead.

'You need to treat me to ice cream for taking me out in the sun today,' she demanded.

'Yes, ma'am!' I bowed in a curtsy while holding the car door open for her.

Crunch, Lift and Bend

The Untold Story of Women and Weightlifting

I t was my cousin Rhea's birthday, and I opted to present her with dumbbells. I recalled a recent discussion in which she had expressed her interest in purchasing them. Although she had always been health-conscious, her dedication to working out had significantly increased over the past year, and she was eager to incorporate weight training into her routine. I believed dumbbells would be the perfect gift for her.

Stunned silence ensued as I unveiled my gift. From Rhea to her mother, none seemed too pleased.

Before we could say anything, Rhea's mother expressed her disapproval. 'Manan beta, girls shouldn't receive such gifts. We understand Rhea is tomboyish and behaves like one of the boys with you all. But this is not acceptable. Can we return it?'

I wouldn't say I was surprised. I had a feeling this might happen and had already guessed the reason, but still, I asked, 'What happened, Aunty?'

'Don't you know? Lifting weights will make women bulky and muscular. Moreover, Rhea is of marriageable age now. We are already trying to find matches for her. A bulky woman is a no-no in the marriage market.'

I stifled a laugh and replied, 'No, Aunty!'

'Oh, I should've known you'd be clueless about this. Here, take it back. If you can't return it, just pass it on to one of your guy pals, please.'

I quickly interrupted her, 'No, Aunty! What I meant to say is that women don't bulk up from lifting weights.[1] It's just one of the many tall tales women have been spoon-fed for years.'[2]

According to a 2018 study, only 20 per cent of women in America engaged in weight training, despite the American College of Sports Medicine recommending strength training twice a week.[3] The reason is quite simple—they didn't want to bulk up or look masculine. That was also why they opted for feminine activities like aerobics, Zumba and the like.

Is it true? Let's find out.

There is absolutely no truth to this theory.[4] In fact, women *should* lift weights for various reasons. Prior studies have highlighted the significance of resistance training for the physiological, psychological and social well-being of women.[5] It can significantly reduce your odds of experiencing back and knee discomfort. Plus, it's like a superhero for your joints, kicking away osteoarthritis pain![6]

'Here, try this,' I offer the dumbbells to Aunty.

'Na na . . . I have severe back pain and knee pain. I cannot do this. It will only get worse!' Aunty promptly interjected.

'On the contrary, this should be your reason to do it! Women are more prone to osteoarthritis, but guess what? Strength training is our secret weapon to keep it away![7]

Let's not forget about other conditions such as type 2 diabetes[8] and heart diseases[9] as well in which weight training also acts as your *suraksha kawach*. And of course, the effect it has on your mood, body image and confidence is simply unmissable![10]

'So, Aunty, you gave me one reason not to lift weights, but I gave you many reasons to do so. I guess I won this round! Now, what do I get?'

'What do you want?'

'How about you join Rhea from tomorrow and start weight training?'

Aunty didn't hesitate for a moment before declaring, '*Ab toh dangal hoga*!' and stretched her palm as Rhea joined hands with her.

Crack, Pop, Oops!

Debunking Exercise Fables

Our quarterly family gatherings were quite the roller coaster. Sometimes we celebrated victories, while other times, we mourned losses. But through it all, our bond only grew stronger. Last weekend's gathering was no exception.

As I sat amid the jovial chaos of a family gathering, savouring the aroma of home-made delicacies and the warmth of familial bonds, the topic of fitness suddenly took centre stage. Ritu Masi animatedly shared her newfound love for Zumba, boasting about her energetic moves and newfound enthusiasm for fitness, especially in her forties.

'I'm absolutely smitten with Zumba. It's such a delight! I eagerly wait for the evening. We switch up the songs daily and it's an absolute blast. It doesn't even feel like exercise, yet it is!' Ritu Masi beamed with joy.

'Zumba? Isn't that too much strain on your joints, especially at your age?' quipped my uncle, Vikram, with a half-concerned, half-teasing smile.

His words echoed with a hint of scepticism, drawing curious glances from the gathering. But before the conversation could veer into the realm of misconceptions, I felt compelled to intervene.

'Vikram Mama,' I chimed in, a playful twinkle in my eyes, 'joints naturally wear down with age, leading to degeneration. However, Zumba or any other exercise is good for your joints. In fact, any form of exercise is![1]

'You see, our joints are designed to move, just like a well-oiled machine. And what better way to keep them in top-notch condition than through regular exercise?[2] I explained, gesturing animatedly for emphasis.

'Exercise, including Zumba, strengthens the muscles around the joints, providing them with crucial support and stability. It also enhances flexibility and promotes better circulation ensuring that your joints remain supple and resilient,'[3] I continued.

Ritu nodded eagerly, her eyes sparkling with newfound understanding. 'So Zumba won't make my knees creak like rusty hinges?' she quipped, earning a round of laughter from the gathering.

'Sure, joints wear out with age—it's nature's little gift to remind us we're not getting any younger. But hey, that's no excuse to become a couch potato!' I reassured her, a smile playing on my lips.

'But my neighbour Kantibhai injured his knees at the gym. He's currently undergoing physiotherapy,' Vikram Mama said, his eyes moving swiftly across the room.

'Getting injured while working out in the gym or lifting weights is a different kind of injury, Mama,' I said. 'And that can also be cured with correct medication and physiotherapy.'[4] (Worried about knee pain and running? Turn to page 207 to find the answers.)

Vikram Mama looked lost in thought, so I nudged him, 'Mama, what are you thinking?'

'A friend has been inviting me to play tennis with him and I kept avoiding him due to this fear,' he confessed.

'Oh, please call him right away and say yes. Start from tomorrow so that the next time we meet, you also have some tennis adventures to share with us, just like Rita Masi's Zumba adventures!' I smiled.

The Tobacco Tango

Chewing Your Way to Trouble

As an Indian doctor in a bustling urban setting, I've seen my fair share of unusual habits and beliefs when it comes to health. One such eccentricity comes in the form of my security guard, Bittu. Now, Bittu is a character straight out of a Bollywood film, with his signature moustache and a knack for storytelling that could rival any seasoned actor's. He was a huge Ajay Devgn fan and that was evident in his haircut and the way he walked.

One day, as I made my way to the clinic, I spotted Bittu in his usual spot near the entrance, his cheeks bulging with what seemed to be an endless wad of tobacco.

Instead of getting into my car, I walked towards him and asked, 'Bittu bhai, you are slowly turning completely into Ajay Devgn, I must say.' And then I made the famous V-shaped hand gesture with two fingers to say, '*Bolo zubaan kesari* (a popular *gutkha* ad that translates to 'say your lips are red')?'

He blushed because he took it as a compliment and returned the gesture.

So I asked further, 'You started eating tobacco after seeing his ads? Or is there any other reason?'

160

'*Sa'ab*, growing up, I have seen everyone back in the village eat this. I don't even remember when I had it first. But yes, it feels good to see Ajay Devgn in the ad,' he responded in Hindi with a smile.

'But what about the harm it causes?' I asked with genuine curiosity.

Bittu, ever the philosopher, looked at me with a twinkle in his eye and paused to spit before replying, 'What harm, Doctor sa'ab? Tobacco is not harmful. Cigarettes and *bidis*, now those are the real villains. And don't even get me started on alcohol—that's poison! But tobacco? It's harmless, I tell you.'

His conviction was palpable in his voice, his tone and even his dialect; I found myself almost swayed by everything he said. Just then, Bittu turned to his right, put two fingers on his lips and let out a long jet of red spit. It hit the wall right across from his cabin, painting it red. I couldn't stand those stains; they were like unwanted guests popping up everywhere—at railway stations, inside trains, in hospital corridors, even in parking lots!

My expression must have been a dead giveaway at this sight, I am sure, as Bittu looked at me, confused.

Gathering my wits, I gestured for him to sit down. 'You are mistaken, Bittu. Chewing tobacco is harmful to your health.'

Did You Know?

Oral cancer[1] ranks as the third most prevalent cancer in India, following cervical and breast cancer.

Chewing tobacco might seem harmless compared to cigarettes and alcohol, but it's far from harmless. In fact, it can cause a whole host of health problems.

Chewing tobacco contains harmful chemicals like nicotine and tar, which can wreak havoc on your body. It can lead to oral cancer, gum disease and even heart problems, not to mention that it stains your teeth and gives you bad breath![2]

Oral cancer is a significant health issue and the main factors contributing to the prevalence of the disease are tobacco, alcohol and betel nut use.[3]

Bittu scratched his head, mulling over my words. 'But Doctor sa'ab, everyone in my village chews tobacco, and they're all fine,' he argued.

I nodded sympathetically. 'I understand, Bittu, but just because something is common doesn't mean it's safe. In fact, chewing tobacco is a major health risk.[4] You're young and have a beautiful family with young children. Why risk your life for such a pointless addiction?'

Bittu fell silent, his usually jovial demeanour replaced by a contemplative expression. After a moment, I said, 'Do you know it is also a punishable offence[5] to spit on the road and in public places? The fine is Rs 5000 or imprisonment and Rs 500 for every day the offence is continued. Now imagine, what if someone from the building complained about you to the government?'

In the span of a minute, his face morphed from denial to shock, then to surprise, and finally settled into a state of helplessness. Bittu found himself scratching his head in bewilderment.

As my phone rang, I made my excuses and stepped away. Walking towards my car, I silently hoped that my words had made some impression on Bittu. If not the fear of death, then perhaps the threat of imprisonment would deter him from this destructive habit.

Microwaves Unmasked

Dispelling Misconceptions

D uring the usual lunch hour at the hospital pantry, the atmosphere is bustling with the sound of people enjoying their meals with colleagues and exchanging stories about their day so far. The air is infused with the aroma of spices, oils and various dishes. Those who haven't brought their own lunch queue up at the canteen counter to place their orders with the canteen attendant. 'Two vada pavs!' someone shouts, followed by, 'And two teas!' In this chaos stands a white microwave in one corner, quietly watching all the visitors.

When I first joined, the area would mostly be deserted. Gradually, more people began utilizing it, but considering the size of the staff, it still remained largely unutilized. As for the reasons behind this, I never bothered to find out, nor did I have any interest in doing so.

This continued till one day when a new colleague named Ankita joined us during lunchtime. As usual, I took out my lunch box, transferred the contents onto a glass plate and was about to put it in the microwave when she exclaimed, 'What are you doing, Doctor? It's not healthy. Please don't eat like this.' Her voice was loud enough for everyone to stop in their tracks and look at us.

I paused for a moment, unable to process what had just happened, and then it hit me: the microwave monster had arrived. With a smile, I placed the plate in the microwave, turned it on and walked back to the table.

Seating myself, I looked at Ankita and asked, 'So what exactly happens to the food to make it unhealthy? Because I'm pretty sure I packed a perfectly healthy lunch this morning!'

Without a moment's hesitation, she launched into an explanation of how microwave radiation annihilates the nutrients, vitamins and all the healthy components of food with its intense heat. According to her, what we're served after microwaving is essentially 'dead' food, unfit for consumption by living beings like us. Her eyes betrayed the genuine fear and concern behind her words.

'Ankita . . .' I interrupted her by holding up my hand, 'what if I told you microwaves are completely safe?'

'I'm not buying it, sir,' she said with a serious expression.

'I'm dead serious, Ankita. The microwave doesn't destroy any nutrients in food.'[1]

Did You Know?

Every electronic device emits radiation[2] and this includes the mobile phones we use, which rank at the top of the list.

The adverse effects of microwave radiation do not directly pose any hazards to human health.[3] You may have heard rumours that it even causes cancer,[4] but let me tell you, that's just not the case.

'Long story short, heating your meal in the microwave is as harmless as watering your plants. After a day of battling office politics, dodging coffee spills, attending to patients and calming their worried families, you deserve the sheer luxury of piping hot leftovers. Trust me, Ankita, the only thing the microwave is radiating is convenience, not radiation.'

Ding! The microwave chimed, beckoning me to retrieve my meal. It seemed that the same bell must have rung in Ankita's mind as well, for I noticed her trailing behind me with her own lunch box in hand.

When I turned to her, she admitted somewhat sheepishly, 'I'm craving something warm for lunch today.'

Blend and Beware

The Dark Side of Meal Replacement Drinks

As I pulled up to Aslam's building, I saw him emerge holding a mysterious crate. My friends in the car started speculating, 'Beer for the road trip, huh?'

But to our surprise, Aslam revealed that the crate was filled with meal replacement drinks.

'Meal substitute drinks? Care to explain?' I asked.

As soon we hit the road, Aslam began his sales pitch about these miracle drinks. 'They're supposed to help me shed those extra kilos. A friend of my uncle's cousin's neighbour lost 20 kilos in a month with these!'

On seeing the questioning look on our faces, Aslam adds, 'I've only just started taking it a few days ago and didn't want to disrupt my routine on this road trip. So here we are!'

These words were enough to launch me into my doctor mode.

Marketed as meal substitutes, these products evade stringent pre-marketing testing and regulations. Consequently, their ingredients remain undefined, lacking quality control or evidence of their efficacy and safety.[1]

Numerous sources highlight the adverse effects of these products, with hepatotoxicity being the most common harmful side effect.[2] These products have also been linked to a range of damaging effects on the liver, varying from minor hepatogram alterations to severe cases of hepatitis necessitating liver transplant.[3] Liver damage often occurs as a result of the use of such meal substitutes and their by-products, as the liver is the primary organ responsible for metabolizing drugs,[4] being the first in line to experience the repercussions and in the most delightful manner imaginable!

'Listen, Aslam, there are no magic potions for weight loss. It's all about a balanced lifestyle, exercise and eating healthy food. These meal-substitute drinks will harm you rather than heal you, bro! Please stay away from these.'

Finally, Aslam seemed to come around. 'You know, Manan, I feel so lost when it comes to health these days. There's so much conflicting information out there.'

'I hear you, Aslam,' I replied, feigning solemnity. 'In fact, I feel so lost right now that I forgot to turn on the GPS while we were talking. And now, we actually are lost!'

'Time to reverse?' Aslam asks.

A bit surprised by his question, I looked at him and he said, 'For both of us?'

Amid laughter, we agreed to ditch the meal replacement drinks and focus on enjoying the road trip with actual food and great company. Aslam promised to see a qualified nutritionist as soon as he was back in town and learn to manage his weight effectively.

Fitness Folly

The Truth About Exercise and Junk Food

'Excellent work with those burpees! Keep that energy up! Take a sip of water and push out one more rep,' cheered my gym instructor.

I took a swig from my water bottle and spotted Aniket across the gym. We'd started our fitness journey together a year ago and followed the same instructor until Aniket disappeared. Assuming he'd switched classes, I didn't think much of it.

'Hey, what's up?' Aniket greeted me as our eyes met.

'Good to see you again! How have you been?'

'Same old,' he sighed, grabbing at his waistline, 'but you look like you've been hitting the gym hard. Spill the secret.' His serious tone caught me off guard.

'Oh, you know, just following the tried and tested formula of a healthy diet, active lifestyle and hitting the gym. No secret potions involved!'

'I too have been sticking to the routine religiously. But check this out.' He pointed to his love handles again.

Then his phone rang—it was his wife, ordering French fries with burgers from McDonalds for evening snacks.

He glanced at me sheepishly. 'It's our cheat day today, so we're indulging in some French fries and burgers for dinner!'

His admission sparked an idea in my mind.

'Let's be real here—how often do you eat out in a week?' I was genuinely intrigued.

'About two or three days, sometimes four on rare occasions,' he admitted. 'But I make sure to balance it out by eating healthy the rest of the time. And I hit the gym extra hard to counteract the effects of all that junk food.'

'So let me get this straight: you're devouring everything in sight and hoping those dumbbells will transform into a magic wand?' I was confused.

The confusion on his face mirrored mine.

'My friend, that is the perfect recipe to stay unfit!' I joked to the rhythmic clinks of weights and the hum of treadmills around us.

He didn't seem to find it amusing, though, so I explained. 'Weight loss is a combination of exercise, healthy food choices and good sleeping habits along with nutrition.[1] Exercise alone has a minimal impact on weight loss.'[2]

He gestured for me to halt and hastily said, 'Just tell me what worked for you. I'll follow it blindly.'

I put a hand on his shoulder and with an all-knowing glance, nodded and said, 'It doesn't work like that, bro! Weight loss strategies should be tailored to each individual by experts.'[3]

Each individual responds differently to various exercises. Assuming that one approach will work for everyone is misguided and not the right approach to fitness.[4] There isn't just one best diet for losing weight.[5] You can never outrun a bad diet. The golden rule is—*diet for fat loss, gym for muscle gain*.

Weight loss can be achieved through healthy living[6] and that is a choice to be made every day, in everything that we do. And believe me, there are no magic tricks. It's all about putting your nose to the grind. Every darn day. Yep, consistency is the secret sauce.

'Every decision is like walking a tightrope between salad bowls and double cheeseburgers. The struggle is real, man!' I pointed towards a guy doing crunches, his face revealing the struggle. Yet, the outcome? Oh, it was definitely making an appearance . . . on his midsection!

'I am cancelling my cheat meals right away and getting back to the grind,' he said, wiping the sweat beads from his face. 'Manan, thank you, yaar! How can I ever repay you?'

'By starting to work out today!' I instantly answered, pointing to the empty treadmill next to us.

'Does burning my heart with these scary stats count as a pre-workout warm-up?'

One look at his face and I knew for sure, the healthy bug had finally bitten him. And this time, it was a lifelong infection.

White vs Brown Bread

A Crumbly Debate

I t was 8.30 a.m. when I hurried to the breakfast buffet, knowing that the seminar would commence promptly at 9. With just a short window to grab a bite, I headed to the restaurant. Upon arrival, I witnessed a small commotion; some guests were expressing their discontent over the absence of brown bread in the buffet spread to the server.

'It's healthier, you should provide it. What's the point of coming to a renowned hotel otherwise?' one person exclaimed. Lacking the time to engage in the discussion, I swiftly filled my plate with some poha and reached for a few slices of white bread. At that moment, the same individual spotted me and ceased his protest.

'Dr Manan,' he addressed me, gesturing towards my badge. 'Yes?' I responded, uncertain of his intentions. 'Don't worry, I've spoken to them. They're arranging for brown bread. You needn't settle for this unhealthy option,' he assured me, eyeing the four slices of white bread on my plate.

'Um, well, it doesn't really make much of a difference . . .' I attempted to explain, but the disbelief on his face mirrored the surprise of finding white bread on my plate.

I approached the table, unwilling to prolong the discussion, when the gentleman, accompanied by a few others, joined me.

One of them queried, 'Did I hear correctly that you believe there's little disparity between white bread and brown bread?'

I nodded in affirmation while continuing to consume spoonfuls of poha.

'How can you possibly say that, Doctor? You must be misinformed,' remarked one of them incredulously.

'It's not me who's mistaken, my friend—it's you,' I retorted with a hint of sarcasm.

'How about you . . .' I gestured towards the individual on my right, 'search the Internet for the ingredients of white bread.' Then turning to the person on my left, I added, 'And you, do the same for brown bread.'

By now, it was clearly evident that two teams had formed. The situation resembled the fastest fingers first round of *KBC* with Amitabh Bachchan, as they all scrambled to get the results before anyone else.

The brown bread results looked like this: wheat flour (atta)—32 per cent, refined wheat flour (maida), yeast, sugar, vital gluten, iodized salt, refined palmolein, preservative, emulsifier, improver, acidity regulators, vitamins and flour treatment agent.

The white bread results looked like this: refined wheat flour, sugar, yeast, edible common salt, edible vegetable oils (palm), soya flour, class II preservatives, acidity regulator, vitamins, flour treatment agent and antioxidant.

They remained puzzled, thrusting their mobile screens with the two results towards me, their questioning stares probing for answers.

'In the ingredient lists, items are listed in descending order of quantity. If you observe, refined wheat flour, also known as maida, is the second ingredient in brown bread as well. The remaining ingredients are identical.' At that moment, it felt as though I had just unveiled a revolutionary insight, only to be met with a silence like Einstein's after he'd made a groundbreaking discovery.

White bread has 70-80 calories while brown bread has 80-90 calories. There is a slight difference in the nutritional value. As white bread is processed, it contains endosperm, which is responsible for its high starch content. Hence, it has lower nutritional value. For brown bread or multigrain bread, the germ and bran stay intact throughout the process and hence it is more nutritional.

For taste enhancement, most of the breads have sugar in some form, like corn starch or high fructose corn syrup. Moreover, many times, malt or caramel is added to give a distinct brown shade to the bread. To opt for a healthier choice, simply seek out whole wheat as the key ingredient. The higher, the healthier!

'Simply put, whether it's white or brown bread, they're basically bread siblings in the grand scheme of things! Neither is healthier than the other.[1] And unless you're indulging in multigrain bread or even the sophisticated sourdough, the white versus brown bread debate is hardly worth the worry!'

I savoured the last morsel of bread and signalled to the waiter for another round. The expressions around me were a whirlwind of shock, disbelief and then pure hunger as they all clamoured for the waiter to bring them white bread too.

Up, Up and Away?

The Truth About Milk Supplements for Children and Their Tall Claims

Assisting patients in achieving optimal health for children is a fulfilling aspect of my profession that I genuinely enjoy. While I do endeavour to unwind from work on weekends, there are occasions when the boundaries between my personal and professional life blur. This occurred a few weeks ago during a visit to my friend Adil's house.

We were meeting after a long time. Our conversations were mostly filling the other in on our lives and our adventures over shikanji and nuts. With the musky smell of khus curtains, the whirring sound of the cooler and the cool air it brought, the comfort of sitting with an old friend felt heavenly.

After a while, our conversation was interrupted by a grocery delivery which was attended by Sheeba, Adil's house help.

She took the bags inside and unpacked them meticulously. We had just started talking again when we heard her lament, 'Oh gosh! Looks like I forgot to order Bournvita and now it is out of stock,' her voice tinged with frustration.

Her distress caught the attention of Adil's mother, who was lounging nearby, engrossed in a soap opera. 'Bournvita?' she exclaimed, her eyes lighting up with excitement. 'Oh, we must get it for Rehaan! All his friends have shot up like bamboo shoots in the rain, and he's still as short as a stump. We can't let him be left behind!'

Adil interjected, 'If not Bournvita, then go for Complan, Horlicks or Boost. Any of them will suffice for Rehaan. They all help children in gaining height.'

I couldn't help but chuckle at the dramatic scene unfolding before me. The age-old Indian belief in the miraculous powers of milk supplements for children to spur height and growth was alive and well in this household. After all, that is what the ads have been promising for decades now!

These words were enough to activate my white coat mode and I was ready to make a difference.

'Sorry to cut in, but I need to share this with you.' I paused for dramatic effect before continuing, 'Bournvita, or, for that matter, any other such milk supplements for children, don't help to increase height in any manner!'

The stunned silence that followed this declaration could have put any good television serial to shame. The only thing missing was the background music of *Dhoom taana na . . . Nanana . . .*

Did You Know?

In 2023, the National Commission for Protection of Child Rights (NCPCR) sent a notice to Cadbury Bournvita[1] for misleading advertisement.[2]

Nutrition plays an important role in growth and development. However, height is primarily determined by genetics.[3] Drinks like Bournvita, Horlicks, Boost and Complan may contain nutrients that support overall health, but they won't magically make you taller. Height is influenced by a complex interplay of genetic factors, hormonal balance and environmental factors.[4]

Sheeba looked crestfallen while Adil's mother seemed reluctant to let go of her belief in the miraculous powers of these milk supplements. Just at that moment, someone in the soap opera screamed, 'Nahi!' with her hands on her ears. *Perfect timing*, I muttered under my breath.

'What do you suggest we do, Manan?' Adil finally broke the silence.

'There are plenty of ways to support your nephew's growth and development without relying on tall tales. Encourage him to eat a balanced diet, get plenty of exercise and ensure he gets enough sleep.' I smiled and turned to Sheeba, 'You can stop feeling guilty about missing it now. Consider it to be a blessing in disguise!'

Sheeba breathed a sigh of relief while Adil's mother looked unconvinced and asked, 'But we can still give it, right? To add some flavour to milk.'

'No, Aunty. It's not as innocent as it appears, even for adding flavour. Let's not forget the hefty sugar levels packed into these kiddie supplements. Always keep an eye on what your little one is munching, especially when it comes to sugar. It can be a real sweet disaster!'

Each of them exchanged solemn glances, maybe pondering who would shatter the silence, when the doorbell rang once more. It was the delivery man, holding a packet of Bournvita in his hand. 'It seems I missed delivering this. It fell out of the packet.'

Almost instantly, all three of them exclaimed, 'Noooo!'

Therapy Unveiled

It's Not Just About Chit-Chatting

One Sunday evening, we had all gathered at my Mama's place for Chai pe Charcha, which is what we called our quarterly get-togethers.

A bunch of us cousins were sitting inside with Nanaji and catching up on life. Amid jokes and stories, we had some great milestones to celebrate. Soon, it was my cousin Ria's turn to speak.

'Well, I have something I need to share,' Ria began, her gaze darting nervously around the table. 'Lately, I've been feeling really overwhelmed with stress, and I think I might need to seek therapy to help me cope.'

Her words hung in the air, met with a mixture of surprise and concern from the rest of us. But before anyone could respond, Nanaji chimed in with a dismissive wave of his hand.

'Therapy? Oh, come on, Ria, therapy and self-help are just a waste of time. If you need someone to speak to, I am here. Why pay a stranger to listen to you?' Nanaji declared, his tone sceptical.

I couldn't help but sigh inwardly at Nanaji's words, knowing all too well the misconceptions and stigma that still surround mental health and therapy in our society. But rather than let his ignorance go unchallenged, I decided to seize the opportunity to shed some much-needed light on the topic and hopefully change a few minds in the process.

'Sorry to butt in like this, but I need to speak. Therapy can be incredibly beneficial for managing stress and improving overall mental well-being,'[1] I interjected, my tone calm yet firm. 'Therapists provide a safe and supportive space for individuals to explore their thoughts and feelings, gain insight into their behaviours and develop coping strategies to better navigate life's challenges.'[2]

As I spoke, I could see the scepticism melting away from Nanaji's face, replaced by a genuine curiosity and interest in what I had to say. So I launched into an impassioned monologue about the many benefits of therapy and why it's far more than just 'talking about your feelings'.

'Therapy isn't just about venting your frustrations or seeking validations,'[3] I explained, my voice growing animated with each passing moment. 'It's about gaining a deeper understanding of yourself, your patterns of thinking and behaviour, and how they may be contributing to your stress or mental health issues.[4] And by working with a trained therapist, you can learn valuable skills and techniques to better manage your emotions, improve your relationships and live a more fulfilling life.'[5]

As my cousins listened intently, I could see the scepticism slowly melting away, replaced by a newfound appreciation for the power of therapy in promoting mental well-being.

I shared my final thoughts, 'I commend Ria for her bravery in seeking help. It takes immense courage to do so, and she's handling it admirably, I must say. As her family and well-wishers, it's our responsibility to stand by her, offer our unwavering support and assure her of our presence. We should regularly check in on her and be ready to lend a listening ear whenever she needs it (read about mental health on page 228).'

Ria, who till then had looked like she was on the brink of breakdown, looked at me and smiled, whispering, 'Thank you!'

The Lone Ranger

Why Your Swimmers Aren't in Danger

It was a weekend getaway to Kapil's farmhouse in Alibaug for his bachelor's party. The party was a gathering of friends and family—all men, of course. We had organized poolside games accompanied by great music and ordered food from our favourite artisanal cafe nearby.

As we wrapped up our pool game, our appetites were sharpened by the arrival of our food. Gathering around the lounge, we eagerly dug into our meal. That's when Rohit, always the instigator, proposed, 'Let's play truth or dare!'

It sounded crazy, but the idea sparked excitement among us. So, with unanimous agreement, we positioned an empty bottle at the centre of the table and gave it a spin. Fate intervened, pointing directly at Arpit, Kapil's sixteen-year-old cousin. Amid cheers and laughter, Rohit posed the inevitable question, 'Truth or dare?' Arpit opted for truth.

With heightened anticipation, Rohit challenged him, 'Tell us one of your deepest, darkest secrets, one you've never shared with anyone.'

Arpit hesitated at first, blushing furiously, but eventually, he confessed, 'I've never masturbated in my life . . .'

The room fell into stunned silence as Arpit's confession hung in the air. Shock and disbelief etched onto our faces, mirroring the range of emotions coursing through the room. Somewhere deep down I knew there was more to this story. Curiosity getting the better of me, I asked the question on everyone's mind, 'But why?'

Arpit's response was swift and resolute. 'A few years ago, when I was twelve, I had been warned about the supposed perils of masturbation by my friends and some seniors at the school. They told us how it could potentially impact sperm count and fertility and also threaten future parenthood. So, I decided not to jeopardize my future with this potential threat. Ever since, I've purposely kept my distance from what I consider to be a serious problem.'

There were some approving nods and some lingering confusion, but I felt compelled to interject. 'Bro, that's not true. Masturbation doesn't have any negative impact on sperm count.'[1]

Despite the well-documented individual, relational and health advantages, masturbation has faced social stigma.[2] Additionally, widespread social stigma and medical misconceptions have frequently portrayed masturbation as harmful to human health, leading to certain apprehensions regarding its acceptability.[3]

Contrary to popular belief, it actually has a few perks. Masturbation enables individuals to explore their sexuality, enjoy pleasure and understand their bodily responses, potentially fostering healthy sexual development, self-esteem and body positivity.[4] Abstaining from masturbation is often suggested as a way to enhance sexual self-control.[5] However, there is no medical evidence supporting this idea.

'And yes, masturbation won't magically lead to hair loss, acne outbreaks or muscle meltdown. Those tales are as imaginative as the bedtime threats from our childhood, like "*So jaa warna* Gabbar *aa jayega!*"'

With every sentence I said, Arpit kept turning redder and redder.

'Manan bhaiya, all this is making me feel stupid, yaar!' Arpit was embarrassed.

'Don't feel that way! We all are learning, bro. All I want to say is that whether to masturbate or not is a personal choice, and neither choice has any impact on our health.'[6]

Kapil asked, 'What do you suggest, Doctor Manan?'

'Listen to your heart, my friend, and do what makes you happy!' I said.

Pulses

The Protein Pretenders Exposed

One sunny Sunday afternoon, I bumped into Karan in our building lobby. After the usual exchange of pleasantries, he couldn't help but notice my gym attire and gym bag.

'Hey, Manan! I've been meaning to ask, which gym do you go to?' he inquired eagerly.

'Oh, I go to the gym down the street. It's pretty decent,' I replied. 'But what about you? I thought you were already hitting the gym.'

Karan's expression turned a bit sour. 'Ah, I quit my old gym. Wasn't getting anywhere with their diet plan,' he confessed.

'Diet plan?' I raised an eyebrow, curious.

'Yeah, they put me on this high-protein diet. I started eating loads of pulses daily. But my body just wasn't responding. And they couldn't do anything about it,' he explained with a hint of frustration and exclaimed, 'I need a place that actually delivers on its promises.'

'Karan,' I said hesitantly, 'pulses are not a great source of protein. They are not enough when compared to our daily requirements. Relying solely on pulses for your protein requirements is not correct.'

The average person typically requires a certain amount of protein per day to support bodily functions, muscle repair and overall health. This daily requirement varies based on factors such as age, weight, activity level and health status.

Now let's scrutinize the protein content of a bowl of pulses. Sure, pulses pack a protein punch, offering around 7 to 9 grams[1] of protein per 100 grams depending on the variety. But let's be real—a single serving is nowhere near enough to meet your daily protein needs.

The minimum protein requirement for an individual typically ranges from 1.2 grams to 2 grams per kilogram of body weight. This means that for optimal health and muscle maintenance, a person weighing 70 kg would need between 84 and 140 grams of protein daily, depending on their activity level and specific health goals.

Let's get real here—7 to 9 grams of protein per 100 grams from a bowl of pulses will never cut it for a 70 kg individual needing 84 to 140 grams of protein daily.[2] Do the maths. You'd have to consume an impractical amount of pulses to meet your required intake. It's simply not practical to rely on pulses alone for your protein needs.

'By this, I don't mean you should jump to non-vegetarian options like eggs and meat. Vegetarian and even vegan diets have plenty of choices to meet your protein needs effectively!' (See page 213 for the various sources of protein for vegetarians.)

'Wow, that's quite enlightening! This new insight is definitely a game-changer. So, based on this information, what dietary choices would you suggest for meeting our protein requirements?' The creases on his forehead were quickly disappearing.

'It's important to complement pulses with other protein sources[3] to ensure adequate intake. Incorporating a variety of protein-rich foods such as dairy, tofu, nuts and seeds, or eggs, lean meats and fish, into one's diet can help achieve a well-rounded protein intake that supports overall health and vitality.'

While there is no single best strategy for weight management,[4] one can keep working on weight management in many ways. The right diet is the first step to this.

Karan sounded thrilled, 'This is really motivating! I feel like heading back to the gym right now. I've been missing my workouts too.'

I smiled, 'You know the saying "*Kal kare so aaj kar, aaj kare so ab*"? So why wait any longer?'

He nodded and gave me a fist bump before rushing home to pick up his gym bag.

The Long and Short of It

Why Size Doesn't Stand Tall in the Bedroom

Fridays typically meant diving deep into reports at work, crunching numbers, analysing data and making observations. So when my friend Rohan called, it was a welcome break from the analytical world I was floating in.

'Hey Ro, what's up?' I chirped into the phone, but his response was far from enthusiastic. 'Hey Manan, how are you doing, man?' As our conversation unfolded, Rohan shared his concerns about his younger brother, Siddharth, who had just finished college and was preparing to go abroad for a Master's degree.

'I don't know where he got the idea that his penis is small, and now he's really worried about it. I tried talking to him a few days ago, but it doesn't seem to have made a difference. His distraction from his studies is really worrying me,' Rohan explained.

'Oh Ro, don't stress out too much. Why don't you bring Siddharth over for a game of FIFA this weekend at my place? I'll have a chat with him,' I suggested, trying to ease his worries.

Fast forward to the weekend and there we were, gathered around the console, ready to battle it out on the virtual football field. With the friendly banter and competitive spirit in the gathering, Siddharth seemed to relax a bit.

'Messi is so short. I wonder why anyone would bank on his football skills?' I commented casually while playing FIFA, making Siddharth and Rohan glance at me.

'Manan bhaiya, Messi is a brilliant player. What has his height got to do with his playing skills?' Siddharth asked.

'Exactly what the size of our penis has got to do with pleasure and arousal!' I paused the game and looked at him.

He stared accusingly at Rohan and then at me. Now that I had his attention, I wanted to talk about it all.

'Siddharth, let me get straight to the point. We've all experienced moments of insecurity about our bodies, especially in this age. For girls, it might be about the size of their breasts, and for guys, it often comes down to their penis size. Men often underestimate their size.[1]

'Speaking as a doctor, I want to emphasize that size really doesn't matter. When it comes to arousal and pleasure, the size of your penis plays no role whatsoever.'[2]

Did You Know?

The average length[3] of an erect penis is between 5.1 and 5.5 inches.

Well-known sex researchers have found that the size of the male penis doesn't actually affect female sexual satisfaction[4] in any significant way. They reached this conclusion after studying how the vagina adjusts[5] to accommodate different sizes of penises.

The key ingredients for great sex can be summed up in three Cs: comfort, compatibility and consent.

I could see the tension easing from his shoulders as my words sank in. It was clear that he had been carrying this unnecessary burden of insecurity for far too long.

'Just think of it like this—would you judge the performance of a football player solely based on the size of their shoes?' I quipped, hoping to drive my point home with a touch of humour.

He chuckled at the analogy, finally starting to see the absurdity of his concerns. 'I guess you're right, bhaiya. Thanks for putting things into perspective,' he said, a hint of relief in his voice.

'I am so glad to see that smile on your face, champ!' Rohan said, holding Siddharth by his shoulders.

'Ah well, guys! Siddharth might be the champ at your home. Here, I am the champ in FIFA. Beat me if you can!' I screamed and turned the game on as we all got back to serious gaming.

Sun's Up, Guns Up

Shattering the Morning Exercise Illusion

ate one evening, as I lounged on my couch after a long day at the hospital, my phone rang. It was Rohan, an old friend from college.

'Hey Manan, we're having a small get-together at my place this Thursday night. Can you make it?' he asked enthusiastically.

I hesitated for a moment. 'Sorry, Ro, I can't. I hit the gym in the evenings, so weekdays are a bit tight for me.'

'Wait, you go to the gym in the evenings?' Rohan sounded surprised. 'But isn't it better to work out in the morning? That's what everyone says.'

I chuckled. 'Well, well, well, Mr Know-It-All! Let me enlighten you with some groundbreaking news: there's no sacred scripture carved in stone dictating the divine timing of workouts. Shocking, I know. Feel free to break the shackles of tradition and hit those dumbbells whenever the mood strikes you. Who knows, maybe midnight push-ups will be the next big trend!'

While we emphasize the importance of exercise for everyone in all age groups, we also need to know that the ideal timing of exercise for health benefits has not been determined.[1]

In simpler terms, there's potential for optimal training response[2] at any time of the day—morning, afternoon and evening.

Rohan seemed intrigued. 'Ha ha ha . . . Really? I never thought about it that way. I've been slacking off on my workouts lately. My schedule's been crazy with all this travelling and mornings are just chaos.'

I nodded understandingly. 'I get it. But listen, it's never too late to get back into it. The key is consistency.'

'Our schedules are hectic, I get that,' I said, acknowledging the constant busy-ness of our lives. 'We might not always be available to exercise at a specific time. But the good news is, it's perfectly fine to work out at any time of the day. The important thing is to stay consistent, considering our busy schedules.'

I continued, 'So if you can squeeze in a 20-minute HIIT workout, go for a 15-minute jog, take a brief walk on the treadmill, or even follow a quick 20-minute dance workout on YouTube—that's great. Don't worry about the clock. If you find a window to exercise, just go for it. What really matters is that you keep moving.'

Did You Know?

The American Heart Association[3] recommends 150 minutes of moderate-intensity exercise per week as sufficient.

This means we don't need to stress about fitting in hour-long workouts every day at the same time. On busy days, you can aim for short workouts. These shorter sessions will add up over time, having a compound effect on your overall fitness.

Rohan sounded determined. 'You're right, Manan. I'm going to make it a priority again. Thanks for the motivation.'

'No problem, buddy. And don't worry about Thursday dinner. I will also be working out that evening!' He chuckled and said, 'Let's plan something for the weekend, when we can all relax a bit.'

With that, we said our goodbyes, and I couldn't help but smile. It felt good to see someone prioritize their health, even if it meant cancelling a dinner plan. After all, what's more important than taking care of yourself?

Sugar Scandal

The Truth About Brown vs White

During a leisurely drive, my friend Karan suggested we make a pit stop on the highway at a nearby tea shop that he highly recommended. It turned out to be owned by an engineer-turned-entrepreneur with aspirations of establishing a chain of tea outlets across India. This cheerful proprietor was eager to share the unique qualities of his tea with us. As we placed our orders, I requested a sugar-free one.

With great enthusiasm, he assured me, 'No problem, sir! I have brown sugar. It's healthier than white sugar.'

As he reached for the brown sugar, I nearly leapt over the counter, exclaiming, 'Noooo!' Four pairs of eyes, including his and the others', glared at me with irritation.

I raised my hands and said, 'I can explain . . .' The tea shop banter came to a screeching halt with all eyes now fixed on me, awaiting my explanation.

White and brown sugar originate from the same crop: sugarcane. So, what makes them different? It is the process.[1] Brown sugar is primarily white sugar mixed with molasses, a sugar-based syrup that gains its colour from extensive boiling, which also produces amino acids and plant pigments.[2] It has a distinct flavour and is made by evaporating and concentrating sugarcane juice.[3]

Brown sugar has a slightly lower calorie content compared to white sugar, but the difference is negligible. Moreover, the levels of minerals in brown sugar are so low that it's not a reliable source of vitamins or minerals.[4] Nutritionally, they are nearly identical. The primary distinctions lie in their flavour and appearance.[5]

'If we follow that flawed logic, then all kinds of sugar are harmful!' the man at the tea stall exclaimed with a mixture of anger and disgust, shaking his head in sheer rebuke.

Before I could reply, Karan interjected.

'I am feeling like Devdas now!' He sounded offended.

'What?' I was baffled at his confession.

'*Babuji ne kaha* coffee *chhod do, sab ne kaha daru chhod do, aaj tumne keh diya chai chhod do . . . ek din aayega jab woh kahenge, duniya hi chhod do*': Karan was at the peak of his dramatic flair (popular dialogue from the movie *Devdas*, modified to 'Father asked me to quit coffee, everyone asked me to quit alcohol, and today, you have asked me to quit tea also. One day they will ask me to quit this world').

I burst into fits of laughter.

The chai shop owner quipped, 'Bhaiya, you're jeopardizing my business with this! Where will us chai vendors end up if even chai is deemed harmful?'

'It is not the chai, it's the sugar. There is no such thing as "healthy sugar". Sugar is harmful whether it is white or brown. Options like Stevia are healthier than sugar. And of course, sugar-free chai is the best way to still have chai and not let it harm your health.'

'Sure? Lock *kar diya jaye*?' Karan's imitation of Amitabh Bachchan from *KBC* was even more comical.

Our eyes met for a moment, silently conveying a message of trust.

The chai shop owner grinned. 'Seems like our *chai pe charcha* has been going on for a while, and the chai has gone cold. Let me brew a fresh batch for all of you. And this time, I'll make it without sugar for you, sir!'

'For us too!' chimed in several voices from the crowd along with Karan. The nods and smiles around me filled me with the hope of conquering the sugar monster soon.

Ashwagandha

The Wonder Herb That Leaves You Wondering

'A-S-H-W-A-G-A-N-D-H-A, and it's a triple word score too!' Aditya pumped his fist before plunging his hands into the bag to draw new alphabets.

We were playing Scrabble and this left me stumped—not the score, but the word.

'That's an interesting word. How did you even think of it?' I had numerous questions.

'Oh! All of us in the family have been taking it for years now. Including my eighty-year-old grandmother,' Aditya responded automatically.

I blurted out, 'That word may have earned you a triple word score, but the havoc that herb is wreaking on your body is a hundred times worse.'

'As in?' Aditya's innocence was mildly disturbing.

'Where do I start?' I was struggling to frame my responses so as to not scare him for life. 'To begin with, the so-called benefits lack scientific backing. They wreak havoc on a multitude of our organs, causing irreparable damage.'[1]

Consumption of Ashwagandha can cause liver injury.[2] It promises to cure everything from a paper cut to a meteor strike but is a habitual promise-breaker. Its effectiveness in treating stress–related conditions, neurological disorders and cancer is not backed by any research.[3] The notion that ashwagandha has significant effects on brain disorders is just another unproven myth floating around.[4]

What's worse is that it can trigger various adverse reactions such as diarrhoea, vomiting, headaches, dizziness and allergic responses,[5] among others. Ashwagandha also can cause complications for pregnant women, people with thyroid conditions, diabetes and auto-immune disorders, or those who are on blood thinners and sedatives. Due to its calming properties, this magic potion can also induce drowsiness.[6]

'And bro, if you're using it to boost your testosterone after buying into any of those fertility tales, believe me, you don't need it.' I hit the final nail in the coffin.

'No way! That cannot be true!' His reaction betrayed his poorly concealed secret.

I was not impressed. 'I think I should start taking oaths like they do in court before talking about anything related to medicine and science. Perhaps people will take me more seriously!'

Then I raised my right hand and started reading the oath aloud, '*Main* Manan Vora, *jo kahunga sach kahunga, sach ke siva kuch nahi kahunga* (oath taken in court, loosely translating to "I, Manan Vora, swear that whatever I say will be the truth and nothing but the truth"). Are you convinced or should I continue?'

One look at his face and I knew he had no answer. So I continued.

'The wonder drug ashwagandha seems to have taken a vow of secrecy regarding its actions and active ingredients when it comes to male infertility treatment.'[7]

'Well, isn't this a shocker! Turns out those wonder pills I've been gobbling down aren't so wonderful after all. Time for a health reboot, I guess!' Aditya got up and fished his phone out of his pocket.

'Are you sharing this on WhatsApp?' I was confused about his actions.

'Not before cancelling my monthly order of ashwagandha with my chemist!' His smile put all my fears to rest.

'And what about the game?' I asked, pointing to the Scrabble board.

'You won it, my friend!' Aditya winked before placing a call on his phone.

I smiled as science triumphed once again.

No Pain, No Gain . . . or Maybe Not?

The Truth of First Workout Struggles

As a doctor, I often face unexpected calls, but this one took the cake. It was an SOS from a distant relative, Deepak, who sounded like he was in the middle of a fitness apocalypse.

'Dr Manan! I can't move! I'm injured!' Deepak's panicked voice blared through the phone.

I tried to calm him down. 'Deepak, take a deep breath. What happened? Did you have an accident?'

'No, no, I just worked out for the first time in ages, and now I can't even sit or turn in bed!'

'Deepak, listen to me. What you're experiencing is completely normal. It's called delayed onset muscle soreness, and it's a sign that your muscles are adapting to the new stress you've put on them.'

'A friend has told me the pain only gets worse. I will stop going to the gym from tomorrow. This pain is too much to bear.' Deepak sounded worried.

'Trust me, it gets better,' I told him.

Delayed onset muscle soreness (DOMS) often occurs after doing new or intense exercises, particularly those involving eccentric contractions (stretching muscles). It's known for causing tenderness and pain when moving. It is believed it's due to small muscle tears and inflammation.[1]

'But it hurts so much, Dr Manan!'

'I know, I know. But trust me, it's temporary. Your body needs time to recover and adapt. It's like breaking in a new pair of shoes—it's uncomfortable at first, but it gets better with time.'

Deepak sounded doubtful. 'Are you sure?'

Since DOMS can disrupt daily activities and athletic performance and discourage beginners from exercising regularly, it's important to understand ways to prevent it.[2]

'Absolutely. The key to overcoming muscle soreness is to give your body time to heal. Rest, hydrate and maybe try some gentle stretching or light exercise to get the blood flowing. Even massaging[3] the painful areas can be helpful. A good warm-up is important. It starts easy and gradually ramps up until you reach your target intensity for the main workout.

'For instance, if you're planning to do chest presses, it's advisable to begin with 5 kilograms and incrementally increase the weight as your body adjusts, rather than aiming for 30 kilograms right away. And most importantly, don't give up. Consistency is the key to seeing results in your fitness journey.'

After some more reassurance and advice, Deepak seemed to calm down. 'Thanks, Dr Manan. I'll give it a shot.'

'That's the spirit, Deepak! Remember, Rome wasn't built in a day. Take it slow, listen to your body and you'll get there eventually.'

As I hung up the phone, I couldn't help but chuckle. Who knew a simple workout could cause such a commotion? But it was moments like these that reminded me of the importance of patience and perseverance in the pursuit of health and fitness.

Vitamin D

More Than Just a Sunny Disposition

Every morning, like clockwork, I'd spot Mr and Mrs More on their deck, basking in the morning sun like a pair of sun-worshipping turtles. Dressed in their finest home attire, they seemed to be on a mission to absorb every ray of sunlight, all in the name of Vitamin D.

But it wasn't until I bumped into them at a society gathering that I realized just how seriously they took their morning sunbathing ritual. 'Ah, there you two are, getting your daily dose of sunshine therapy,' I quipped, trying to stifle my amusement.

With a look of utter conviction, Mr More nodded. 'Absolutely! Gotta keep those Vitamin D levels up, you know?'

Suppressing a smirk, I couldn't help but intervene. 'Well, isn't that just sunshine-tastic! But did you know there are easier ways to get your Vitamin D fix, even without turning into human solar panels? You don't just have to count on the sun!'

Their puzzled expressions were almost comical as I launched into my explanation. 'You see, while sunlight is indeed a great source of Vitamin D, it is recommended to absorb 5 minutes of sunshine[1] from 9 a.m. to 1 p.m. on a clear day. If it is cloudy, then 10 minutes and 20 minutes if it's heavily overcast.'

Did You Know?

In addition to causing sunburn, sunlight also leads to other biological processes such as skin ageing, weakening of the immune system and changes in skin cell structure.[2]

Sunlight significantly impacts the production of vitamin D3. When it's produced in the skin and exposed to sunlight, it quickly breaks down into different substances that can be harmful.[3] Also, too much sunlight exposure is linked to various health issues like skin cancer.[4] So it's important to be cautious.

Many food items are a great source of Vitamin D. The best non-vegetarian sources of Vitamin D include fatty fish, eggs, liver and other organ meats. The vegetarian options include milk, butter, margarine, mushrooms and breakfast cereals.[5]

Over lemonades and baked samosas, I shared with them the wonders of fortified foods and Vitamin D-rich delights like fish, eggs and mushrooms. All the while I was mentally drafting a letter to the sun, politely requesting it to tone down its UV rays for the sake of my sunbathing neighbours.

'You know, it's a good idea to get tested for vitamin D levels once a year,' I mentioned. 'And if you're deficient, it's worth consulting your doctor about taking some supplements.'

As we debated the merits of sunshine versus salmon, Mr More couldn't help but crack a smile. 'Well, it looks like our long Vitamin D escapades are officially on hiatus, dear,' he quipped, earning an eye roll from his equally enlightened wife.

With a collective sigh of relief, we bid adieu to their sun-soaked mornings and embraced the idea of exploring new, less skin-scorching activities to kickstart their days.

Treadmill Tales

Jogging Through the Knee Mystery

As I wrapped up my workout at the gym, feeling the familiar post-exercise endorphin rush, I overheard a heated discussion near the treadmill area. Curiosity piqued, I sauntered over to see what the commotion was about.

There, I found Kunal, a regular at the gym, engaged in a debate with the trainer.

'I will not do it!' He adamantly refused to step on the treadmill, citing concerns about his knees.

The trainer tried to reason with him and explained the benefits of cardio workouts but Kunal wasn't having any of it.

'Listen, I've heard horror stories about treadmills wrecking people's knees. I refuse to risk it,' Kunal declared defiantly.

Now, as a fitness enthusiast and a doctor, I couldn't help but intervene. 'Hold on there, Kunal! Let's not jump to conclusions,' I interjected, drawing their attention.

Kunal turned towards me, clearly surprised by my interruption. 'Dr Manan, what are you doing here?' he asked, puzzled.

'Saving you from knee-jerk reactions, it seems,' I replied with a grin. 'Look, the fear of treadmills damaging your knees is just a myth. In fact, regular cardio exercise like running on a treadmill can actually strengthen your knees and improve joint health.'[1]

Kunal raised an eyebrow sceptically. 'But I've heard stories, Doc. People claim their knees start aching after using the treadmill.'

I chuckled, shaking my head. 'Let's blame it on anecdotal evidence! Listen, Kunal, each body is different, and it's essential to listen to your own body. But science tells us that when done correctly and gradually, treadmill workouts can actually reduce the risk of knee injuries.'

The trainer nodded in agreement, chiming in, 'That's right. Proper form, warm-up exercises and gradually increasing intensity are key to reaping the benefits of treadmill workouts without straining your knees.'

Kunal seemed to ponder this but wasn't convinced. 'But I've heard running is bad for the knees and can lead to arthritis.'

I couldn't help but smile before explaining how wrong he was.

Running doesn't make knee osteoarthritis symptoms or knee problems worse. It actually helps prevent general knee pain.[2]

I explained, 'Moreover, running on a treadmill is safer because its belt acts as a shock absorber, making it gentler on the joints compared to pounding the concrete outdoors. All I would recommend is to invest in a good pair of running shoes. This way you can prevent knee injuries and protect your joints during workouts.'[3]

Kunal seemed to digest this information, his expression shifting from scepticism to curiosity. 'So you're saying I've been avoiding the treadmill for no reason?'

'Exactly!' I exclaimed, glad to see my words sinking in. 'It's all about understanding the science behind the exercises and debunking those pesky fitness myths.'

With a newfound sense of determination, Kunal finally stepped onto the treadmill, a hint of excitement in his eyes.

'And as you run, remember to have only one thing on your mind!' I cautioned Kunal.

'What?' Kunal voiced the trainer's thoughts.

'Fire on the mountain, run, run, run . . . It will help you run faster!' I gave my golden advice to all runners, just to prove that health and humour always go hand in hand.

Udderly Untrue

Dispelling Myths About Fruits and Milk Together

I have a bit of a love-hate relationship with social gatherings. Sometimes I'm really into them, and at other times they just drain me. It's not that I don't enjoy interacting with people, I do, but it's not always my favourite thing to do.

Last Wednesday, for example, I found myself at a social gathering, not because I wanted to be there, but because I felt like I had to. You know, social etiquette and all that. The problem was that I didn't know anyone at this gathering, and that made it even more difficult to muster any enthusiasm.

As I reached for a refreshing mango milkshake at the social gathering, I heard a voice cautioning me, 'Are you sure you want to mix milk with fruits? It could lead to digestion issues, you know.'

Surprised, I turned to see who had spoken. It was a fellow guest, a gentleman sipping on a glass of plain water. 'Oh, really?' I responded, raising an eyebrow. 'Are you a doctor or a nutritionist?'

'No, not at all,' he admitted. 'But I read it in one of those WhatsApp groups I'm part of. You know how it is with these health tips circulating everywhere.'

Suppressing a chuckle, I introduced myself, 'Well, I'm Dr Manan, and actually, there's no scientific evidence to support that claim.'

His eyes widened in surprise. 'Oh, you're a doctor? Well, I didn't know that. But I've heard it so many times, I just assumed it was true.'

'It's understandable,' I replied with a smile. 'But in reality, there's no evidence to suggest that mixing milk with fruits causes digestion issues. Many traditional Indian dishes like fruit salads with curd or milk-based desserts like mango lassi and fruit custard are enjoyed without any problems.'

In fact, fruits and curds are both considered healthy foods. Fruits are low in calories and packed with antioxidants and fibres, which are good for your digestion. Yoghurt is also rich in nutrients like protein, calcium and vitamins. It contains helpful bacteria that can improve gut health. When you eat fruits and curds together, you get a mix of probiotics, protein and essential nutrients, which can all work together to keep you healthy.[1]

He nodded thoughtfully, clearly intrigued by the new information. 'I guess you learn something new every day,' he remarked.

'Absolutely!' I agreed. 'And that's the beauty of science—it's always evolving, and we're constantly learning new things.'

As the conversation shifted to other topics, I couldn't help but feel amused by the situation. It was a reminder of how misinformation can spread easily, even in today's age of technology.

Later, as I enjoyed my mango milkshake without a care in the world, I couldn't help but appreciate the simple joys of life—good food, good company and the occasional opportunity to bust a myth or two.

In the end, it was just another light-hearted moment in a social gathering, but it served as a reminder of the importance of questioning what we hear and seeking out reliable sources of information.

I don't know how the next social gathering will be, but I definitely know that the next time someone brings up a health tip from a WhatsApp group, I'll be ready to set the record straight once again!

Protein Prowess

Unmasking the Meat-Free Muscle Makers

It was a typical evening in Mumbai, and I was out with my friends at our favourite restaurant, indulging in some good food and lively conversation. As we settled into our seats and scanned the menu, I couldn't help but notice the surprised look on one of my friends' faces.

'Manan, aren't you a fitness freak?' he asked with a hint of disbelief. 'I've heard you're really conscious about what you eat and work out religiously. How come you're still a vegetarian?'

I couldn't help but chuckle at his question. 'Well, I guess I'm just breaking stereotypes,' I replied with a smirk, taking a sip of my black coffee. 'But seriously, being a doctor, I'm well aware that you can absolutely meet your protein needs on a vegetarian diet.'

The question of whether vegetarian diets can meet protein requirements has long been a controversial topic in the field of nutrition. 'Where do you get your protein from?' is a standard question vegetarians and vegans are routinely asked.[1]

Figure 1: Protein intake (gm/day) in the Adventist Health Study 2[2]

He raised an eyebrow, clearly intrigued. 'Really? But don't you need meat for protein?'

'According to a study, the protein consumption of lacto-ovo-vegetarians and vegans closely resembled that of fish-eaters, semi-vegetarians and non-vegetarians.'[3]

'You cannot be serious!' He was astonished.

I shook my head, continuing my explanation. 'Not at all! There are plenty of vegetarian sources of protein that are not only nutritious but also delicious. Take lentils, for example. They're packed with protein and are a staple in many Indian dishes. And then there's tofu, which is incredibly versatile and can be used in everything from stir-fries to smoothies.'

As I spoke, I gestured to the menu, pointing out various vegetarian options that were high in protein. 'And let's not forget about chickpeas, nuts, peanut butter, cottage cheese, seeds, Greek yoghurt, beans, legumes and quinoa,'[4] I continued. 'These are all excellent sources of protein that can easily be incorporated into a vegetarian diet.'

My friend's expression softened as he listened, nodding along with my words. 'Wow, I never knew that,' he admitted. 'I always thought you needed meat to get enough protein. Thanks, bro, this conversation was so helpful.'

I grinned, feeling satisfied that I had cleared up the misconception and signalled the waiter to bring us some lentil soup, when he interjected.

'Make that two, please!'

As I looked at him with curiosity, he responded, 'Soup *pine ka*, gym *karne ka*, tension *nahi lene ka... majaa ni* life. What say, Doc?

We shared a laugh as we dug into our meal, enjoying the camaraderie and the newfound understanding. After all, knowledge is power, especially when it comes to making informed choices about our health and well-being.

Water Wisdom

Pouring Cold Truths on the Standing Ban

Last week marked my friend Rahul's birthday, so I decided to call him up as per my tradition with all my buddies.

He answered the call almost immediately.

'Hey man, what's up?'

His usual greeting cheered me up as I wished him, 'Happy Birthday, Rahul!'

We continued chatting but suddenly, I heard a loud shriek in the background, followed by a few seconds of silence.

'Bro, are you okay?' I blurted out.

'Umm, yeah . . .'

'Phew! I got worried for a second. What was that?'

'I had just entered my house and was thirsty. So I drank from a bottle lying nearby.'

'Okay, and . . .?' I was still clueless about the situation.

'I was standing while drinking the water!' he exclaimed. 'Ma saw me and got livid. She is worried I will damage my knees with this habit of mine. She has warned me so many times!' His guilt-ridden voice was a clear giveaway.

'Hey buddy, I get it, we've all heard some wild stuff, but worrying about your knees while sipping water standing up? That's next-level! Trust me, your knees won't throw a fit over a water-drinking stance. And let's get real here— water's not staging a hostile takeover of your joints! It's just doing its thing, sliding into your bloodstream like a smooth operator. I mean, who's got time to sit down every time they're thirsty?'

I paused for a moment before continuing, 'Water's your body's best friend, and it couldn't care less about your posture. Your body's not going to throw a tantrum over how you sip water.'

You might have heard about the infamous Ayurveda advice about not drinking water while standing. Well, let me tell you, there's no scientific evidence to back that claim. Water is your trusty companion, ready to hydrate you whether you're sitting or standing. And let's just say, science sips water from a different cup!

After my brilliant comeback, there was a silence so long I thought the call had dropped.

'Rahul?' I decided to check on him after what felt like an eternity.

'Huh . . . yes . . . you're sure you are not joking, Manan, right?'

All through my school and college years, my reputation had preceded me: sarcasm and jokes were my trademark. It was a given that anyone who had known me for that long wouldn't take my words at face value.

'Of course, Rahul. This is not a joke.'

'I am putting your call on speaker. Can you say this again? I want my mother to hear this.'

I reiterated everything I had mentioned earlier about drinking water while standing and patiently explained to his mother that there was no reason for concern.

His mother let out a sigh of relief and expressed her gratitude towards me. She swiftly handed the phone back to Rahul, claiming she had some groundbreaking revelations about water-drinking techniques to share with her WhatsApp squad.

We chuckled for a bit, exchanging tales of other health-related conspiracy theories floating around before agreeing it was time to hang up.

'Well, Rahul, if you ever need someone to vouch for your knee's water-drinking preferences, you know whom to call! And don't let the naysayers be your health guide.'

We both laughed in unison.

The Sweet Truth
Crushing the Fructose Fiasco

It was one of those balmy evenings in Mumbai when the humidity felt like a wet blanket, and the only thing on my mind was something refreshing to cool down. So I found myself at a local eatery with a bunch of friends, seeking respite in a plate of fresh fruits.

As I dug into the juicy watermelon slices and sweet mango chunks, Roy, a beefed-up friend of my friend, raised an eyebrow and commented, 'Hey Manan, I expected you to know better. Don't you know that fructose from fruits is just as bad as any other sugar? It's all about that sugar rush, you know.'

'That's ironic, because I expected you to know better too, bro,' I said while taking a bite of dragon fruit, and added, 'Because what you said just now is a classic example of "Tell me you know nothing about health and fitness without telling me you know nothing about health and fitness!"' I replied with a grin.

'Huh?' another friend, Siddhu, gasped.

I quickly wiped my mouth with a tissue and smiled, 'Fructose may have its downsides, but not all fructose is created equal. Excessive consumption of added sugar can wreak havoc on your health, but the sugars present in whole fruits are packaged differently. They come bundled with fibre, vitamins and minerals which mitigate the negative effects of sugar.'[1]

My friends exchanged puzzled glances, clearly intrigued by the impromptu nutrition lesson they were receiving at our humble eatery.

'Let me break it down for you,' I said, leaning in as if about to reveal the secrets of the universe.

I held three fingers up to demonstrate what I was saying next.

'There are various types of sugars, glucose, fructose and sucrose among them. Glucose is what your body runs on, so it's essential for energy. Fructose is found naturally in fruits and is metabolized differently from glucose. And sucrose? Well, that's just a fancy name for table sugar, which is a combination of glucose and fructose.' I paused to see their reaction.[2]

My friends nodded along, absorbing the information like eager students in a classroom.

'Now, here's the kicker,' I said, lowering my voice for dramatic effect. 'It's not the sugars found naturally in whole foods like fruits that you need to worry about. It's the added sugars that sneak their way into processed foods and beverages that are the real troublemakers. Those are the ones linked to a whole host of health problems, from obesity to heart disease.'[3]

A look of realization spread across my friends' faces as they connected the dots. 'So you're saying it's not the fruit itself that's the problem, but rather the way sugars are added to other foods?' one of them ventured.

'Exactly!' I exclaimed, feeling a sense of triumph at their newfound understanding.

If you look closely, almost all the snacks and drinks in the market contain sugar,[4] from tomato ketchup to ready-to-eat noodles—sugar is an active ingredient in each one of them.

'So the next time you're craving something sweet, reach for a piece of fruit instead of that sugary snack bar. Your body will thank you for it!' I winked at Roy, reminding him of the snack bar he had just some time back as we were on the way to this place.

The sheepish look on his face followed by the all-knowing smiles of my friends was a sign that the sugar monster had finally been defeated.

'Excuse me . . .' Roy signalled the waiter, 'Can you also get me a plate of fresh fruits please?'

I gave him a slight nod, showing my appreciation for making the right move.

Virginity

More Than Just a Red Herring

I t was the weekend and we were embarking on a trip to Lonavala with friends. Three of us planned to pick up our fourth friend, Sahil, before heading directly to the highway. The early hours of the morning promised lighter traffic and a refreshing breeze. We sacrificed some sleep to ensure an early departure, eager to avoid traffic jams caused by mass family weekend travel plans.

On reaching Sahil's building, I promptly called him and let the phone ring once. That was our sign for him to come down. As I sat in the car with my friends, waiting for Sahil to join us, the atmosphere was light and filled with banter. My friend, Rohan, was scrolling on his phone, seemingly lost in the depths of the Internet. Suddenly, his brows furrowed and he let out an exasperated sigh.

'What's got you so worked up, Rohan?' I asked, curious about his expression.

He turned his phone towards me, displaying an advertisement for hymen reconstruction surgery. 'This is so unfair, man,' he exclaimed. 'Now we'll never know if the girl we marry is a virgin or not.'

'You are joking, right?' I asked, but the serious expression on his face told me otherwise.

Rahul chimed in in agreement. 'Yeah, it's ridiculous! How are we supposed to trust anyone these days?'

'Yaar, I cannot believe this. We are in 2024 and you are talking as if it is the 1980s!' I was livid.

Their blank faces told me they were clueless about what I was saying. So I clarified, 'The idea that a woman has to be a virgin is wrong on so many levels.'

'Virginity is a social construct, and it's unfair to judge someone's worth based on outdated notions. It's important to challenge societal norms and educate ourselves about these matters,' I said. 'In any case, the idea that a woman has to bleed the first time she has sex is anyway incorrect,' I added.

Rohan raised an eyebrow. 'What do you mean?'

The belief that virginity can be determined by the presence of an intact hymen[1] is a common misconception. The hymen[2] is a thin membrane that partially covers the opening of the vagina.

'Contrary to popular belief, an intact hymen is not a reliable indicator of virginity. In fact, the hymen can tear or stretch for a variety of reasons other than sexual intercourse.'[3]

Rahul was getting irritated. 'Like what?'

'Like physical activities such as horse riding, gymnastics or cycling,'[4] I explained. 'Even inserting tampons or undergoing a gynaecological examination can cause the hymen to tear.'[5]

Not all women experience bleeding the first time they have sex.[6] This notion stems from outdated cultural beliefs and misinformation. Bleeding during intercourse is not a reliable indicator of virginity and the absence of bleeding does not mean a woman has had previous sexual experiences.[7]

Engrossed in this discussion, we failed to notice when Sahil joined us in the car and only realized it when he spoke. 'Absolutely. We shouldn't be placing so much emphasis on a woman's virginity. What matters most is mutual respect, trust and open communication in any relationship.'

Rohan sounded philosophical when he said, 'You know, Manan, every time we have these discussions, I'm left in awe of the miracles of science and nature, even the magic happening right inside our own bodies. It's like our bodies are secret agents with hidden superpowers, and we're just here, clueless about most of it!'

Saying this, he reached out for a cigarette from his pocket and tried to light it.

That's when I added, 'Oh, and let's not forget the things we do know but conveniently choose to ignore! Like smoking. The packet boldly screams "I kill" but hey, who has time to listen to a mere warning label, right? Even when smoking is not only harmful for the smoker but also for others around the smoker (read more about passive smoking and its ill effects on page 145).'

Dairy Drama

The Truth of Curd's Alleged Crimes Against Your Stomach

My cousin Radha paid us a long overdue visit, reigniting memories of our childhood adventures. As we sat down for a hearty lunch, curds were served alongside our meal. Engrossed in our lively conversation, I absent-mindedly extended a bowl of curd to Radha, only to be met with a startled expression. 'No, Manan,' she declined with a hint of offence, 'I cannot afford any stomach bugs or cold infections right now. I have a lot of travel planned in the coming weeks. Curd is off-limits for me right now.'

'Oh, did a doctor advise you that?' I was genuinely concerned.

'No, no. I haven't needed to see a doctor yet. But this is the age-old advice we have been practising ever since I can remember,' she answered matter-of-factly.

I put the bowl on my plate and started singing, '*Sardi khasi na* malaria *hua, yeh gaya yaaro isko*...myth myth myth mytheria *hua* (a popular Hindi film song modified to "No cold or cough, this person has been infected with mytheria")!'

Radha exclaimed, 'Thanks for ruining my childhood favourite song like this. Now this will haunt me forever!'

'Just like your words will ring in my head!' I retorted.

'What?'

'That curd can cause stomach issues and also lead to cold . . .' I smiled while putting a spoonful of curd in my mouth.

She looked at me with a puzzled expression.

'Eating curd does not cause cold or digestion issues,' I explained.

Curd is a wholesome food enriched with the benefits of probiotics. It contains a harmonious blend of essential nutrients vital for our body and well-being.[1]

In addition to this, curd provides an abundant supply of B vitamins, proteins and calcium. As a result, it serves as an optimal dietary choice for individuals with sensitive digestive systems, especially young children and the elderly.[2]

It is also helpful in dealing with insomnia[3] and enhancing the immune response.[4]

'I call curd the magical stress-buster! Just imagine, stress hormones trembling in fear as curd swoops in like a superhero to transform them into feel-good hormones. If only life were as simple as a bowl of curd!'

Radha's expression shifted from one of confusion to that of enlightenment.

To lighten the mood, I broke the trance. 'Aap convince ho gaye ya main aur bolu?'

She promptly recognized my impersonation of Kareena Kapoor from *Jab We Met* and waved her hand in exasperation. 'The same old *filmi* Manan, you haven't changed at all!'

'Some things are good as they are,' I smiled, 'just like this bowl of curd.' And so saying, I offered her a bowl of curd, which she accepted not just readily but gleefully.

Occasionally, dispelling age-old myths simply requires a dash of science and a pinch of logic.

Teenage Mood Swings

A Roller Coaster or a Deep Dive?

The day was bright and sunny with a gentle breeze wafting in through the open windows of our modest living room.

Dad's friend, Sharma Uncle, visited us in the afternoon. The conversation soon turned to more serious matters as Sharma Uncle broached the topic of parenting teenagers with a hint of concern in his voice.

'You know, my son is going through a rough patch these days,' Sharma Uncle began, his brow furrowed with worry. 'He's always moody and irritable, and I just can't seem to figure out what's bothering him. But I suppose it's just a phase all teenagers go through, right? Just hormonal fluctuations and a desire for attention, nothing to worry about.'

As I listened to Sharma Uncle's words, a pang of concern tugged at my heartstrings, prompting me to speak up and offer some much-needed insight into the complexities of adolescent mental health.

'Well, Sharma Uncle, while it's true that teenagers can experience mood swings due to hormonal changes, it's important not to dismiss poor mental health as just a passing phase,' I replied, my tone gentle yet firm. 'Adolescence is a time of immense change and upheaval, both physically and emotionally,[1] and it's not uncommon for teenagers to struggle with their mental health during this period.'

As I spoke, I could see a flicker of understanding in Sharma Uncle's eyes, prompting him to lean in closer, eager to learn more about the nuances of adolescent mental health.

'Adolescence is a time of immense vulnerability, with teenagers facing a myriad of pressures and challenges from all sides,' I continued, my voice soft but resolute. 'From academic stress and peer pressure to issues at home and struggles with identity and self-esteem, the list of potential triggers for poor mental health is endless. And while mood swings are a normal part of adolescence, they can also be a red flag for more serious underlying issues such as depression, anxiety or even suicidal thoughts.'[2]

The mention of the word suicide stunned everyone. As the weight of my words settled over us like a heavy blanket, I could feel the gravity of the situation sinking in, prompting Mr Sharma to nod solemnly in agreement.

'It's true, Manan. I never realized just how much teenagers can be affected by poor mental health,' he admitted, his voice tinged with regret. 'But what can I do to help my son? How can I support him through this difficult time?'

With a reassuring smile, I reached out to Sharma Uncle, offering him words of encouragement and guidance as we embarked on a journey to navigate the complexities of adolescent mental health together.

'Well, Uncle, the first step is to create an open and supportive environment[3] where your son feels comfortable discussing his feelings and seeking help when needed,' I suggested, my tone gentle yet firm. 'Encourage him to talk openly about what he's going through and reassure him[4] that he's not alone[5] in his struggles. And remember, even the smallest sign of distress should not be ignored—it's always better to err on the side of caution and seek professional help[6] if needed.'

As our conversation stretched into the afternoon, I could sense newfound hope and determination blossoming within Sharma Uncle as he vowed to do whatever it took to support his son through his struggles with mental health.

While leaving, Sharma Uncle hugged me a little longer than usual and in that hug, I could feel his gratitude and relief.

Prescription Perils

The Painkiller Adventure Unravelled!

On Wednesday evening, after wrapping up work, I made a quick stop at the next-door pharmacy to grab some shampoo and conditioner sachets for my upcoming travels. As I browsed, a man approached the pharmacist, Dineshbhai. He seemed like your average thirty-year-old—educated and well-dressed. Let's call him Mr X.

'Please give me a painkiller for body aches,' Mr X requested.

While Dineshbhai went inside to fetch the medicine, I struck up a conversation with him.

'Hi, I'm Dr Manan. If you don't mind, could I see your prescription?' I asked politely.

Mr X seemed slightly irritated. 'Why do you need my prescription? I don't have one anyway.' His tone was defensive. Just then, the pharmacist returned with the requested medicine.

I glared at Dineshbhai and snapped, 'You're aware it's against protocol to dispense painkillers without a valid prescription, aren't you?'

With a determined glint in my eye, I decided to use this moment as an opportunity to educate both of them about the potential risks of self-medication.

'Taking painkillers, or for that matter any medication, without proper guidance from a doctor is ill-advised. Such medicines can pose serious risks to your body,' I explained.

'But they are all available at medical shops in any neighbourhood. How can such openly available medicines be harmful?' Mr X was now losing his cool.

'Did you know there is no list of medicines defined as OTC drugs[1] (over-the-counter drugs, which can be sold without a prescription) in Indian law? Moreover, painkillers are strictly categorized as prescription drugs under Schedules H and H1. So when a pharmacist sells painkillers to a customer without a valid prescription or based on their own advice, it's illegal and considered an over-the-counter sale of painkillers.'[2]

With those words, I glared angrily at Dineshbhai, who swiftly retrieved the medicine strip from the counter and stashed it back into his drawer.

'You see,' I continued, 'medication should never be taken lightly. In fact, overuse of medication can lead to a whole host of issues, including dependency, adverse side effects and even the masking of underlying health conditions.'

The room fell silent as my words sank in, the gravity of the situation dawning on both of them.

'All you need to do is consult a doctor before taking any medication. Whether it's a headache or body ache, a doctor can provide the right diagnosis and treatment plan tailored to your specific needs.' Saying this, I placed my hand on Mr X's shoulder, trying to convey the seriousness of the situation and willing him to understand.

Mr X nodded in agreement, understanding in his eyes. 'Thanks, Dr Manan,' he said earnestly. 'I never realized how serious it could be. From now on, I'll make sure to consult a doctor before buying any medicine.'

'Sorry, Mananbhai, I won't give painkillers without prescriptions anymore. Please don't file any complaints against us,' pleaded Dineshbhai, his eyes filled with genuine concern.

After Mr X hurriedly exited the shop, showering me with thanks, I glanced at Dineshbhai and cheekily gestured with a V sign from my eye to his, signalling, 'I've got my eyes on you! No funny business, alright?'

To that, Dineshbhai simply nodded and touched his ears.

Cramping Your Style

Breaking the Taboo on Period Pain

It was Friendship Day and we had a grand plan to gather at our favourite eatery in town. Even the pouring rain couldn't dampen our spirits as we shared live locations on our way through the downpour. Most of us had arrived, but I noticed Pooja was conspicuously absent. Concerned, I tried calling her, only to find her phone switched off. Panic surged within me—this was entirely out of character for Pooja.

'Has anyone heard from Pooja?' I asked my friends, hoping for some news.

Almas chimed in, 'Oh, she must have gotten her periods today. We usually attend yoga classes together, but she missed them this morning. She does this only when she is on her period.'

'But her phone is switched off!' I remarked.

'Her cramps are next-level unbearable. They knock her out so bad that she needs to take the day off and cocoon herself with a hot water bag all day. Painkillers are about as effective as sprinkling fairy dust on her agony. It's no wonder she's gone off the radar today. With our gathering on the cards, one of us would've definitely reached out, pleading for her to join. And she is just too embarrassed to talk about this!' Almas said while settling down in her seat.

Sid, looking puzzled, remarked, 'I don't get it. Period pain is normal. I have seen my mother and sister function normally even in their periods. Why would Pooja turn her phone off and miss yoga just because of that?'

Leaning back, I took a deep breath before responding, 'Well, Sid, it's not as simple as you might think.'

Did You Know?

Approximately one in every four women undergoes distressing menstrual pain, which often necessitates medication and leads to absenteeism from studies or social activities.[1]

A milder form of menstrual pain is known as normal menstrual cramps.[2] A severe type of menstrual cramp is known as dysmenorrhea, which is akin to cramps and is characterized by a dull, throbbing ache originating from the lower abdomen.[3]

While some level of discomfort during periods is normal, severe pain and disruption in daily activities could be a sign of underlying disorders like endometriosis, PCOS or PCOD. These conditions can cause intense pain and heavy bleeding, making it difficult for individuals to carry out their usual routines. It's important to recognize when period pain goes beyond the norm and seek medical advice.[4]

Almas exclaimed in surprise, 'The next time I see her, I'm going to insist that she consult a doctor. She's been enduring this for far too long!'

'But those TV ads make it seem so simple!' Sid exclaimed, looking perplexed.

With a chuckle, I replied, 'Don't even get me started on those misleading ads for period products. They make it seem like a walk in the park when, in reality, it's more like a roller coaster ride. Instead of scaring us straight, these ads are on a mission to convert us into die-hard cricket fans by bleeding blue!'

'After listening to this, I can't even fathom the pain women endure every month,' remarked another friend.

'We may not be able to imagine, but we can strive to understand, and that's what we ought to do,' I advised as all of them looked at me with seriousness and concern.

I glanced at their serious expressions and couldn't resist a playful jab. 'That'll be 5000 rupees. Cash or kind, take your pick,' I deadpanned. They exchanged puzzled looks until I clarified, 'My consultation fee. Payment accepted in the form of settling the bill.'

Sid caught on and signalled to the waiter, a knowing smile on his face.

Coffee Chronicles
The Only Guilt-Free Crime Scene

In a world filled with questionable choices, there's one beverage that stands accused, tried and toasted—coffee. Considered to be one of the most widely consumed beverages across the world, it is known for its rich aroma and flavour.

Coffee is made from roasted and ground coffee beans. It derives its dark colour from the coffee beans. The darkness and the richness of its taste depend on the roasting and other elements mixed with it. This includes chicory, hazelnut, chocolate and many others. The taste ranges from bitter to acerbic.

Ever wondered why a sip of coffee feels so rejuvenating? It is the caffeine coursing through your veins, a shield against fatigue, a magical elixir banishing drowsiness to the nether realms. Caffeine is a bioactive molecule found in plants like green coffee beans and cacao beans. It quickly enters the bloodstream through the small intestine after ingestion, reaching its peak concentration within 30 minutes on average.[1]

Coffee can be easily called the fuel on which millions of human bodies function across the globe, but it is still

237

considered unhealthy. It has faced allegations of causing sleepless nights, jittery nerves and even addiction. Black coffee, the unsung champion of this saga, has often been blamed for crimes it didn't commit. But fear not, coffee enthusiasts, for the truth is as bitter as your favourite black brew.

Coffee consumption is safe.[2]

But . . .

If you are someone whose daily number of cups of java consumed is directly proportional to the number of hours you work, then you are in for a surprise (caution: not a pleasant one, of course!).

Consuming up to 400 mg/day (one to four cups per day) of coffee is considered safe for an individual.[3]

> **Bonus Tip:** Savour your coffee without the companionship of sugar and milk, because who needs extra baggage?

Now, let's go on a caffeinated journey through the hallowed halls of scientific studies and look at it closely.

Coffee consumption can reduce the risk of endometrial and liver cancer.[4] It even helps substantially reduce the risk of liver cirrhosis.[5] The diseases on this list are many and includes Parkinson's, type 2 diabetes, breast and prostate cancer and cardiovascular diseases.[6]

This potion has the power to keep the much-dreaded D word, a.k.a. depression, away too.[7]

The benefits of coffee might need a separate book altogether, but you get the drift. In short, coffee is a beverage so profound that its very essence defies containment. To confine its essence within the pages of a book is to attempt to leash a comet—a commendable, if not entirely sane, pursuit.

Remember, the secret is to keep it to three cups a day—because health, much like humour, is best served black. Forget those calorie-loaded concoctions; let your coffee be as pure and untamed as your unfiltered thoughts. Sorry Starbucks, black coffee just stole the show!

Face-Off

The Great Exfoliation
Hoax Unveiled

ast weekend, I was visiting my friend Shilpi. As we sat in the living room catching up, her younger sister Neha burst through the door, fresh from a shopping spree.

Neha was excited, 'Hey, Di! You won't believe what I got! I bought this amazing exfoliating cream. The beauty expert at the cosmetics shop recommended it and she said it works wonders!'

'Oh, really? What's so special about it?' Shilpi was curious.

Neha shared, 'It's supposed to make your skin super smooth and glowing. You have to try it, Shilpi! I'm sure you'll love it.'

Shilpi said, 'Hmm, I don't know. I've never used an exfoliating cream before.'

Neha was insistent, 'Come on, Di, live a little! It's going to be fun. We'll have a little spa day at home!'

I couldn't help but chuckle at her earnestness. 'Neha, you don't need to worry about using that. Exfoliation isn't as necessary as you think it is.'

Her brow furrowed in confusion. 'But everyone says it's important for removing dead skin cells and keeping the skin looking fresh and youthful.'

I motioned to her to sit on the couch next to Shilpi, preparing to debunk this common misconception. 'Yes, I know that's a popular belief, but the truth is, our skin has a natural process of exfoliating and renewing itself. The outermost layer of our skin, known as the stratum corneum, sheds dead skin cells on its own to make way for new ones. This process happens continuously, without the need for external exfoliation.'

Shilpi and Neha exchanged curious glances.

I further continued, 'Continuous exposure to ultraviolet (UV) light results in skin photodamage,[1] the primary culprit behind external ageing[2] caused by environmental factors. Strategies for managing photodamaged skin encompass various approaches such as moisturizers and exfoliants. While numerous treatments exist to counteract this damage, their effectiveness is yet to be fully validated,[3] and they may lead to undesirable side effects.'[4]

Neha's eyes widened in surprise as she listened intently to my explanation. 'So you're saying I don't need to use this cream?'

'Exactly,' I confirmed with a nod. 'In fact, excessive exfoliation can sometimes do more harm than good. It can strip away the skin's natural oils and disrupt its delicate balance, leading to dryness, irritation and even inflammation. Plus, certain exfoliating ingredients, like abrasive scrubs or harsh chemicals, can cause micro-tears in the skin and make it more susceptible to damage.'[5]

Neha lamented, 'Skincare is all so confusing!'

Sensing her distress, I suggested, 'Let me book you an appointment with a dermatologist next week. It is always better to explore skin-related treatments under their guidance to avoid damage.'

Neha's face immediately lit up with joy, and she exclaimed, 'Leave it to you to sprinkle logic and science on the most nonsensical situations and actually make them make sense!'

Calcium Quest

Beyond the Milky Way for Kids' Health

I t was a lazy Sunday afternoon when my phone rang and I saw Rohan's name flashing on the screen. 'Hey Rohan, what's up?' I answered, curious to know what had prompted his call.

'Hey Manan, we finally bought our dream home! You have to come over for the housewarming party this weekend!' Rohan exclaimed, excitement evident in his voice.

'That's fantastic news, Rohan! I'd love to come,' I replied, genuinely happy for my friend.

As we chatted about the upcoming party, I couldn't help but overhear some commotion in the background. It sounded like Rohan's wife, Priya, was engaged in a rather animated conversation with someone.

'What's going on over there?' I asked, unable to contain my curiosity.

Rohan let out a sigh. 'It's Priya and Aarav. She's trying to get him to drink his milk, but he's refusing again.' Aarav was Rohan and Priya's five-year-old.

I chuckled at the familiar scene. 'Bro, don't remind me of the milk struggle days,' I said sympathetically.

Rohan laughed. 'Tell me about it. We've tried everything to get him to drink his milk, but he just won't budge.'

'Well, you know, Rohan, while milk has traditionally been a major calcium source, it is not the only source of calcium for a child,'[1] I said.

Rohan sounded intrigued. 'Really? But isn't milk supposed to be essential for their growth and development?'

I explained, 'While milk does provide essential nutrients like calcium and vitamin D, there are plenty of other sources of calcium[2] that Aarav can consume if he doesn't like milk.'

Rohan was now curious. 'Like what?' he asked and then quickly added, 'Wait, I will put your call on speaker.'

Soon thereafter, I launched into an impromptu lecture on calcium-rich foods, listing alternatives to milk. 'There's yoghurt, cheese, tofu, green leafy vegetables like spinach and even fortified foods like cereals and orange juice,' I rattled off.

Even soy milk and other plant-based beverages, such as those derived from almonds, are great options.[3] Nuts and seeds, particularly almonds, sesame and chia are also abundant sources of calcium.[4] Finger millets, also known as ragi, locally contain the highest amounts of calcium.[5]

Rohan and Priya listened intently as I outlined the various options available to them. 'So, you see, there's no need to force Aarav to drink milk if he doesn't like it,' I concluded. 'As long as he's getting enough calcium from other sources, he'll be just fine.'

A sense of relief washed over Rohan and Priya's voices as they realized they didn't have to engage in the milk battle anymore. 'Phew, that's such a huge weight off our shoulders!' Priya exclaimed.

I grinned at the other end of the line.

'Thanks, bro!' Rohan told me.

'All that is fine. Just ensure there are no milk desserts at the party . . .' I added.

'Why?'

'Well, it's not just Aarav who hates milk!' I sheepishly confessed.

Gym Buffs-Turned-Fluffy Puffs

The Truth of Muscle Conversion

Karanbir, a school friend whom I hadn't heard from in what felt like ages, reached out to me. A straightforward and easy-going fellow, he was known for his love of fun and had propelled his family business to new heights since he'd joined it a decade ago. As we caught up on a video call, I couldn't help but notice the exhaustion evident in his appearance—the bags under his eyes and the swollen face spoke volumes about his fatigue and burnout. Concerned, I inquired, 'Are you okay, dude? You look tired.'

Karanbir proceeded to explain how he was expanding his business, which required frequent travel across the globe. Constantly shifting time zones and short trips left him with little time to acclimate to the differences, disrupting his workout routines for over six months. He lamented that his diligently built muscles were now slowly turning into fat due to these circumstances.

I replied, 'Let's start with the congratulations on your business expansion. I have no doubt that you'll excel in this venture, just as you always have. Now, on to the second matter—I completely understand the hectic lifestyle you're experiencing and its challenges. But bro, those muscles won't be turning into fat anytime soon.'

Muscles and fat are two distinct types of tissues, composed of different cells and structures. Muscles cannot magically transform into fat, nor can fat miraculously morph into muscle. They are metabolically and functionally separate entities in the body.[1]

When you stop exercising regularly, muscle loss occurs. This leads to a decrease in muscle mass through a process known as muscle atrophy.[2] On the other hand, fat gain results from an imbalance between calorie intake and expenditure, not from a direct conversion of muscle tissue.[3] Changes in muscle mass, whether gained or lost, can impact overall metabolism, movement, eating habits and breathing.[4] These are important signs you need to look out for.

'So, if you're noticing a few extra pounds after hitting the pause button on your workouts, don't blame your muscles. It's just simple maths: less calorie burn plus the same old calorie intake equals a delightful little surplus!' I concluded with a smile.

'Oye Manan, *chak de phatte veere*! *Dil jeet liya* . . .' Karanbir exclaimed, his face reflecting his joy. 'I cannot tell you how much this was bothering me!'

'The next time you're in India, you owe me a coffee. That's the fee for this consultation.' I laughed, adding, 'Shall we also have a race like old times and see who wins?'

'Now that's some motivation to get back to working out in whatever way I can between my travels. I must maintain my winning streak at all costs.'

And just like that, it felt like the good old days, with Karanbir's familiar smile gracing his face once again.

Grains of Truth

The Real Scoop on Rice and Weight Management

For centuries, the narrative has been that rice is the culprit behind weight gain. If shedding pounds is the goal, rice is marked as the enemy. Rice enthusiasts face public scrutiny and ridicule for their love of those fluffy, white pearls.

But have you ever wondered if these claims have more holes than a slice of Swiss cheese? Well, today we're your trusty cheese slicer, ready to uncover the truth!

P.S.: *If biryani is your kind of love, get ready to fall head over heels for this too!*

There's no scientific evidence linking weight gain to white rice.[1]

Rice serves as the staple energy source for almost half of the global population, making it crucial for nutrition and health on a significant scale. In Asia, many farmers cultivate rice, rendering it a cost-effective choice for their own consumption. Does asking people to avoid eating it completely sound fair?

No! However, before that, let's understand the reason behind this claim.

White rice is 80 per cent starch and has a high glycaemic index.[2]

A high glycaemic index is the reason behind a sudden spike in blood glucose levels. Foods with high glycaemic index adversely impact the liver. This is the reason people living with diabetes or chronic liver disease are asked to avoid it.

Brown rice and other rice substitutes have a low glycaemic index, making them a perfect replacement for white rice.[3] The sawdust-like charm notwithstanding, though.

Is giving up on white rice the only option for diabetics and liver patients? It's a big fat NO to that!

Hold on to your forks and spoons, for there's an aromatic twist—a solution for devoted white rice enthusiasts who've been reluctantly steering clear.

Prepare the rice, but resist the temptation to indulge right away. Instead, cool it down to a minimum of 4°C and let it chill for a full 24 hours. Then, reheat and savour it the following day. This process ensures your system digests rice slowly, with lower glucose spikes in your blood.[4]

Food with a low glycaemic index is a healthier option for many reasons.[5] This way, you can savour white rice without worrying about those pesky sugar spikes and carb overload.

So, who's ready to spice things up with a biryani bash today?

Choco-Hoax

Unwrapping the Truth About Chocolate's Romantic Powers

I t was Christmas, and the five of us were on our way to visit Mrs Pereira, our beloved English teacher from school. This was a tradition we followed each year except for a few, when life had taken us away from Mumbai. Mrs Pereira's birthday fell soon after Christmas, and this year was her first birthday without her husband after his death eight months ago.

We wanted to lift her spirits. Sudhanshu was behind the wheel, while Rehaan made sure we hadn't forgotten anything.

'Flowers?'

'Check.'

'Scented candles?'

'Check.'

'Books?'

'Check.'

'Gift card?'

'Check.'

'Chocolates?'

'Check.'

Rehaan asked and I responded quickly.

All of a sudden, Mayank raised an eyebrow, questioning our choice of gift. 'Why chocolates? Isn't it a bit odd to give them to a teacher?' he wondered aloud.

I was taken aback, as were the others. 'As far as I know, she's not diabetic. And besides, these are dark chocolates. Even if she has developed diabetes recently, which we're not aware of, these are still a safer option than store-bought sweets loaded with processed sugar!' I explained, trying to reassure Mayank.

'Bro, chocolates are known to be aphrodisiacs. They're more suitable as gifts in romantic relationships, not for a teacher,' Mayank explained.

Now it was my turn to be shocked. I immediately asked Sudhanshu, 'How long till we reach?'

'Google Maps is showing twenty-three minutes,' he quickly responded.

'Great, we have enough time for a quick science class, my buddies. Let's start . . .' I clapped my hands to get their attention and started.

'Due to the instant energy boost and increase in stamina that chocolate provides upon consumption, it's no surprise that its effects have earned it a reputation as an aphrodisiac.[1] But that is not the case.'[2]

'No yaar, I can vouch for this fact. Chocolates do act as an aphrodisiac,' Rehaan confessed sheepishly.

I interrupted him, 'Allow me to explain, bro. Chocolates contain a chemical called phenylethylamine. Phenylethylamine is known to increase blood pressure and heart rate, enhancing sensations and blood glucose levels.[3] This acts as a stimulant as it triggers endorphins in the brain. Endorphins are responsible for making us feel happy as they can change our mood instantly. Some other things endorphins also do are increase the heart rate, raise the blood pressure and increase the heartbeat. All of this also happens when we are excited.'[4]

'Come on, Manan. It's all the same!'

'Nope, it is not same-same, but *alag-alag*,' I clarified and added, 'Chocolates are not an aphrodisiac,[5] milk supplements for children don't help them increase their height and the Earth isn't flat!' My bold declaration was met with stunned silence (read about milk supplements and their claims on page 176).

Though none of them said anything, the looks on their faces combined with sly smiles did reflect enlightenment.

Just then, Siri announced, 'Your destination has arrived.'

I saw Mayank grab the chocolate box, step out of the car and walk towards her building. In my heart, I knew the chocolates were just fine, and once again, science was the guardian angel saving the day.

Breaking a Sweat with Taboos

The Truth About Period Workouts

One weekend, my wife and I were window shopping at a nearby mall when we bumped into her friend Sara. We were gym buddies and for the last few days, we had not seen Sara at the gym.

We were pleasantly surprised to see her, and while talking, my wife asked her, 'Haven't seen you in a while at the gym. Is everything okay?'

Sara nodded,' Oh yes! It's just that time of the month. So I avoid exercising during that time. Will be back at the gym on Monday.'

My wife and I reacted together, 'Sorry, can you come again?'

Sara raised an eyebrow. 'I don't exercise during my periods. Because . . . well, I've always been told that women shouldn't exercise during their periods. It's not good for your health, you know?'

'No, Sara! That is not true,' I said, loud enough to be audible over the noise in the mall.

That's when my wife motioned for us to move to a corner and sit at a cafe table to talk.

While sipping our lemonades, I continued the discussion.

'So, as I was saying,' I said dramatically, 'working out during your period is not only acceptable but beneficial. It's like a natural remedy for those dreaded cramps and mood swings.'[1]

Sara's eyes widened in surprise. 'Really? I had no idea.'

'Absolutely,' I continued. 'Exercise releases endorphins, which are basically your body's happy pills.[2] Plus, it's a great excuse to wear those funky workout leggings and pretend you're a superhero fighting off evil cramps.'

Sara burst out laughing. 'I never thought of it that way!'

If you're dealing with mood swings or anxiety, exercising can be a great remedy. It can also help alleviate headaches, back pain, cramps, muscle soreness, fatigue and even breast tenderness.

Moreover, there was a study conducted on this in which it was found that individuals who refrain from physical activity experienced lengthier menstrual periods, heavier flow and increased levels of fatigue and pain compared to those who did not avoid physical activity.[3] Premenstrual depression[4] is a common symptom among all who menstruate. Working out is a great way to keep those ghosts of depression away.

'Any specific type of exercises you recommend?' Sara was curious.

'You can actually do all types of exercises. The point is to keep moving!' I responded and added, 'The first few days can be really uncomfortable, especially if you tend to bleed heavily. That's why it's important to focus on gentle movements and exercises during this time.'

Many women find that exercising feels harder during this time. So exercises that are usually moderately difficult might feel much more challenging.

Dos and Don'ts While Exercising on Your Periods

Dos

1. Listen to your body.
2. Go for a light walk or jog.
3. Try low-intensity strength training, yoga, Pilates or any other low-intensity or low-volume workout you feel capable of.

Don'ts

Avoid extremely high-intensity or extremely high-volume workouts.

'Bottom line,' I concluded, 'continue exercising, but dial down the intensity, especially if you're feeling fatigued. Vary your workouts, take extra time to recover and honour what you're capable of.'

'And remember, it's okay to just rest if nothing works for you,' I said, giving her a reassuring nod.

'Oh gosh! I cannot imagine the number of days I have wasted by using this as a reason to not work out.' Sara regretted it.

'It is never too late to start working out!' my wife added.

'Exactly,' I said, nodding sagely. 'So next time Aunt Flo comes knocking, don't hide under the covers. Embrace the power of exercise and show those cramps who's boss!'

Sara immediately picked up her bag and said, 'I will see you guys, gotta go!'

We both must have looked shocked as she further explained, 'Don't want to wait till Monday to get back to the gym!'

We raised our lemonades to her as Sara dashed the door.

Damp and Dangerous

Exploring Wet Hair's Health Impact

One morning, while I was waiting for the elevator, I heard my next-door neighbour Shruti calling out to me. 'Please wait for me, Manan. I am running super late,' she exclaimed, hastily grabbing her sandals.

Just as she was about to dash out the door, her mother's voice boomed from within, 'Not again, Shruti! You're leaving with wet hair once more. I've had enough of this, young lady. You're twenty-five years old and still haven't grasped the simplest of things. Going out with wet hair is the root cause of your persistent sinus issues all these years. Come back here this instant!'

I could sense Shobha Aunty's frustration without even seeing her; her tone said it all. Shruti hesitated, coming to a halt mid-step. By then, Shobha Aunty had reached the door, checking if Shruti was still lingering.

Shruti began to plead, 'Mom, I'm already running late. Can we not do this today, please?' Shobha Aunty's face flushed with a spectrum of colours, from pink to red to maroon, in a matter of seconds. It was clear their argument wouldn't be settled anytime soon. Sensing the impasse, I decided to step in.

'Hello, Aunty. How are you?' I greeted her.

'Oh, Manan, you're a doctor, aren't you?' she replied. 'Why don't you say something to her? She never listens to me. She's young and naive, thinks it's okay to play around with her health at this age. But she doesn't realize how all of this catches up with you as you grow older.'

'Indeed, Aunty. I have something to share with both of you,' I began, clearing my throat. 'The idea that wet hair causes sinus or cold is actually a misconception.'[1]

Their actions froze, and all activity ceased as they fixed me with accusatory stares. Aunty likely thought Shruti had put me up to this, while Shruti probably suspected the same.

'I can explain . . .' I said and shed some more light on this.

Sinusitis is an infection caused in your upper respiratory tract.[2] The most common reasons for sinus complaints are viral infections, allergies, smoking and dental infections,[3] among other reasons. Blaming your innocent wet strands for everything from tension to migraines is really taking it a bit too far. Because, clearly, they have nothing better to do than to plot against your well-being!

Aunty tried to butt in, insisting, 'It must be the weather. We're in summer, so it won't affect her . . .' But I swiftly intervened, countering, 'Nope, the weather has absolutely nothing to do with it. Going out with wet hair in cold weather does not cause sinus issues.'[4]

Shobha Aunty did not seem to be very pleased, so I added, 'Well, isn't that a relief? Your body temperature isn't about to burst into a Bollywood dance number just because it's sunny outside!'

As soon as I said this, Aunty's expression shifted, and she smiled. Seeing her, Shruti also heaved a sigh of relief, and I realized that the tension had dissipated.

'Now that we've settled the case against wet hair, Your Honour, may Shruti be excused for her meeting?'

A retired judge, Shobha Aunty immediately said, 'Case dismissed!' Hearing this, Shruti and I dashed towards the elevator.

Double Trouble

The Condom Conundrum

Gathered around the familiar table of our favourite café, my friends and I savoured the warmth of friendship amid the aroma of freshly brewed coffee. As we exchanged stories and shared laughter, the conversation took an unexpected turn, veering towards a topic that was both sensitive and significant.

'So, guys, remember I was telling you about my friend's unexpected pregnancy?' Priya, one of my closest friends, began, her tone tinged with concern. 'Well, it turns out they were using condoms, but still ended up pregnant. Can you believe it?'

Instantly, a ripple of disbelief swept through our group, mingled with a tingle of apprehension. As the gravity of Priya's revelation sank in, murmurs of sympathy and concern filled the air, punctuated by a chorus of questions and conjectures.

'But how is that even possible?' Rohan, always the pragmatic one, chimed in, his brow furrowed in confusion. 'I mean, aren't condoms supposed to be foolproof?'

Before anyone could respond, another voice piped up from the opposite end of the table, eager to share their two cents on the matter. 'Well, I never take chances when it comes to protection,' Arjun declared, a self-satisfied grin spreading across his face. 'I always use two condoms, just to be safe. Better safe than sorry, right?'

Rohan added, 'Best version of *hum do hamare do* in 2024 I could have ever thought of!'

Everyone giggled at this joke but I felt a surge of apprehension wash over me, coupled with a nagging sense of responsibility to set the record straight. With a gentle cough to garner their attention, I prepared to dispel the misconceptions surrounding double condom use, armed with facts and a touch of humour.

'Actually, Arjun, that's not quite how it works,' I began, my tone laced with a hint of amusement. 'Contrary to popular belief, using two condoms simultaneously can actually increase the risk of breakage and slippage rendering them less effective in preventing pregnancy and sexually transmitted diseases (STIs).[1]'

As my friends exchanged puzzled glances, I seized the opportunity to delve into the intricacies of safe sex practices, adopting a light-hearted yet informative approach to drive home my point.

'You see, condoms are designed to provide a barrier between the penis and the vagina, preventing sperm from entering the reproductive tract and reducing the risk of STIs,[2] I explained, my gaze sweeping across the attentive faces of my audience. 'However, when two condoms are used together, the friction between them can cause them to rub against each other, increasing the likelihood of tears or punctures.'[3]

A collective gasp of realization rippled through the group, prompting me to press on with my impromptu lesson on sexual health and safety.

'Furthermore, using two condoms can create a false sense of security, leading to complacency and a lapse in judgement,'[4] I continued.

It's important to remember that condoms are most effective when used correctly and consistently, with just one condom providing adequate protection when used according to the manufacturer's instructions. According to WHO, a condom provides 98 per cent protection[5] against unplanned pregnancy.

'With that being said, it's wise to keep more than one condom handy. This ensures that if one condom breaks or slips off during sex, you have another one available to use,' I said and added, 'And that would be the perfect version of hum do, hamare do in 2024! What say, Arjun?'

The nods I received were a sign that all was well in the condom world for now.

Plant-Based Plunders

Exposing the Vegan Health Hoax

Our group of friends was planning to get together for lunch and various venue options flooded the WhatsApp group chat. Suddenly, Aarav piped up, asking if any of the venues had vegan options, mentioning he had recently adopted a vegan diet.

Surprised by his announcement, I hesitated before responding. 'Choosing your food preferences is completely a personal choice,' I began, 'but it's worth noting that vegan diets can sometimes lead to health concerns.'

His response came almost immediately, brimming with curiosity. 'What do you mean? I have read that veganism is healthier. Moreover, some of my favourite celebrities follow this diet. How can it be unhealthy?'

I said, 'Well, my dear friend, a vegan diet could lead to physical and mental health problems because its restrictive nature often results in the body not getting enough essential vitamins and nutrients.'

Sticking to only vegan food items could lead to deficiencies in essential nutrients like vitamin B12, iron, calcium and omega-3 fatty acids.[1] Vegans tend to experience more mental health issues,[2] which can affect their overall quality of life negatively. Veganism can also lead to health problems, such as issues with the nervous, skeletal and immune systems, and blood disorders due to possible nutrient deficiencies.[3]

Slowly, reactions ranging from ☺ to 💀 started appearing in the group. I was waiting for Aarav to respond, but perhaps he was too stunned to do so.

I nodded sympathetically, understanding his confusion, and typed.

'Well, Aarav, I'm not aiming to terrify you,' I continued typing, 'But let's be real: just because something's trendy or has a celebrity endorsement doesn't automatically make it healthy. Always consult a nutritionist or a reputable doctor to grasp its full impact on your health.'

I reiterated, 'And don't forget to listen to your body. Do regular tests and if something doesn't feel right, it's always best to consult a professional.'

After a long silence, Aarav first liked my messages and then responded, 'Thanks, Manan. I guess I have a lot to learn about this whole vegan thing. It's not as simple as I thought.'

'No problem, Aarav. Just remember, it's all about finding what works for you and your body. And hey, if you ever need any more advice, you know where to find me,' I said, adding a mobile phone emoticon.

'So, it's SodaBottleOpenerWala then?' a friend asked.

To which Aarav responded instantly, 'Yes!'

And soon, pictures of Parsi delicacies ranging from dhansak to lagan nu custard flooded the group as each tried to recommend a dish.

Seed of Doubt

Decoding Papaya Seeds

Amid the midday munching madness, I found myself diving into the depths of social media, only to stumble upon a gem of wisdom: *Papaya seeds—the ultimate contraceptive*!

None of the medical books I had studied to become a doctor taught me that Mother Nature's pantry held the key to family planning. As I chuckled away, Sheetal, a medical student interning with us, strolled in with a curious look, demanding to be let in on the joke. Debunking myths in lunchtime banter sure is a delight!

'First things first, let's set the record straight—papaya seeds have been wrongly tagged as the secret abortion potion. Time for a reality check—in low quantities, papaya seeds do not help guarantee the elimination of unwanted pregnancies.'[1]

She maintained a questioning gaze, urging me to carry on.

'It's a popular belief that munching on papaya seeds can kickstart your menstrual cycle. But there's no medical proof for this old tale. When these seeds took a spin in the lab with our rodent friends, the results were . . . well, let's just say, not so great. A series of uterus troubles leading to period disruption ensued.[2]

'And the misery train isn't slowing down! Brace yourselves, because munching on these seeds can play havoc in the men's department too. Yep, you heard it right—papaya seeds can cause complete loss and damage of the sperm in men.[3]

'Believed to be great at reducing menstrual cramps, they actually do quite the opposite.[4] In extreme cases, they can even lead to serious uterus damage.'

Sheetal's expression shifted shades, but I persisted until I had voiced everything.

'Well, rumour has it that these tiny black pearls even moonlight as a fantastic detoxifying agent. If detoxification is the goal, then our body is naturally equipped to do so. Balance in life is good and that can only be achieved through a healthy diet, a good sleep routine and an active lifestyle. Not by consuming papaya seeds to balance our hormones.'[5]

Sheetal sheepishly retrieved a small packet of papaya seeds from her lunch bag and her face contorted in a guilty expression.

'Oh gosh, Sheetal! No, you can't be having that. Did you know that papaya seeds contain compounds that can mess with your gut?'[6] I asked in alarm.

She gaped in astonishment.

'Yes, it's like inviting trouble to your digestive party. And let's not forget the delightful aroma—or lack thereof. Ever had a spicy lunch date or a reunion feast with a friend, thinking you're in the clear, only to surprise everyone with some unpleasant and unplanned sound effects afterwards? Pretty funny, unless your partner or friend was there to witness the unexpected spectacle!'

'Doc, I still didn't get the joke!' Sheetal confessed.

'The joke is on us, Sheetal,' I added, taking a spoonful of curds from my bowl. 'These tiny seeds boast a robust collection of plant chemicals known as isothiocyanates. These compounds have the potential to harm DNA and induce organ damage, paving the way for the development of cancer.[7] This can even lead to food poisoning[8] in some extreme cases. Who said health cannot be an adventure?'

'Whew, Doc, talk about dodging a seed-shaped bullet!' The relief on her face was clearly visible now.

Then, with dramatic flair, she chucked the packet into the nearest bin like it was a hot potato.

'Remember, the smallest things can pack the biggest surprises—and not always the good kind,' I quipped as we shared a chuckle.

Challenging Conventions

Temple Tours and Time of the Month

As my aunt and her family settled into our Mumbai home for their visit, I couldn't wait to show them around the city. One of the first places on my list was the Siddhi Vinayak temple, a must-visit for anyone coming to Mumbai. Excitedly, I announced my plan to take them there.

But to my surprise, my sister-in-law hesitated and then sheepishly confessed, 'Um, Manan bhai, I can't go to the temple. You see, I'm on my period.'

I chuckled at the absurdity of the comment. 'What do you mean you can't go? Who told you that?'

She looked uncomfortable, clearly embarrassed to discuss the topic. 'Well, it's considered inauspicious to enter a temple during menstruation. It's better to avoid it.'

I couldn't let this misconception slide. 'Oh, come on! Believing in this now is like believing in unicorns, Bhabhi.'

Menstruation is a natural process. For years, it has been shrouded in taboos and myths, often excluding women from various aspects of social and cultural life. These cultural beliefs surrounding menstruation affect the emotional well-being, mindset, lifestyle and health of everyone who menstruates.[1]

I saw her relax a bit, but she still seemed unsure. So I continued my tirade against menstrual taboos.

In our country, menstruation is still culturally perceived as unclean and impure. Before a woman is permitted to resume her family and daily responsibilities, she is often required to undergo a 'purification' ritual. However, from a scientific perspective, menstruation occurs due to ovulation and the shedding of the endometrial lining following a missed chance of pregnancy. Hence, there appears to be no logical basis for the belief that menstruating women are impure.[2]

Numerous girls and women face restrictions in their daily activities solely because they are menstruating. The foundation of this myth lies in cultural perceptions of impurity linked with menstruation. There's also a belief that menstruating women are unhygienic and dirty, leading to potential contamination of the food they handle or prepare. However, scientific studies have not demonstrated that menstruation is a cause of food spoilage as long as basic hygiene[3] practices are followed.

'Avoiding certain food items, skipping exercise and refraining from washing hair during periods[4]—it's like dementors decided to crash the party and drain all the happiness out of women's lives! Have you ever thought about why women are being punished for something that occurs naturally?'

By now, my aunt and everybody else in the house had gathered around us.

'All in all, menstruation is simply a natural biological process and young girls and women should recognize that their ability to conceive is a direct result of this biological function. By that logic, when giving birth is a good thing, so is menstruating.[5]

'Thanks, Mananbhai. You have opened my eyes today!' Bhabhi said.

'Yes, but God's eyes are closed now!' I retorted.

'What do you mean?' Everyone was puzzled.

'I mean, it is time for the gods at the temple to sleep and hence it will be closed. We cannot go now.'

'Ah!' Bhabhi slapped her forehead and quickly added, 'Let's keep that for tomorrow. Today, I will treat you to my special aamras puri at lunch as a treat. But before that, I will first wash my hair.' Saying this, she rushed inside as everyone nodded in approval.

Up in Smoke

Debunking the High Hopes of Marijuana

The Mumbai rains painted a picturesque scene for those residing outside the city, but for those within its bounds, they were synonymous with chaos and inconvenience. A fortnight ago, I found myself caught in the downpour while out with friends. By the time I was dropping off my final companion, the rain had escalated to a torrential downpour. I opted to seek shelter at his place until the rain subsided.

As I lounged on the cosy couch of my friend's living room, the pitter-patter of rain against the windowpane provided a soothing backdrop to our lazy afternoon. With no signs of the downpour letting up anytime soon, we found ourselves embracing the comfort of indoor activities, opting for a laid-back session of board games to pass the time.

My friend's younger siblings Rahul and Riya had some friends over. Chattering and laughing, they decided to spice things up with a game of Never Have I Ever. As the game unfolded, revealing a delightful array of quirky confessions and hilarious anecdotes, I couldn't help but marvel at the infectious energy of youth.

However, amid the light-hearted revelry, a seemingly innocuous revelation sent a ripple of concern coursing through the room. 'Never have I ever tried marijuana,' declared Riya, her voice tinged with a hint of mischief.

Instantly, the jovial atmosphere took a sombre turn as murmurs of disbelief and teasing laughter echoed in the room. 'What? Seriously, Riya? You're missing out, girl!' exclaimed one of their friends, prompting an enthusiastic chorus of agreement from the group.

'It is a once-in-a-lifetime experience!' someone said.

'Let's plan a trip to the mountains this summer with Riya!' quipped another.

Riya's face was a gamut of emotions as she heard all of them and was still confused. Slowly, as the noise subsided, she managed to ask, 'But isn't it unhealthy?'

I was relieved someone saw sense and jumped into the conversation. 'Yes, Riya! You are absolutely right. Marijuana may seem harmless, but it can have serious consequences for your health and well-being.[1]

'You see, marijuana contains psycho-active compounds that can alter your perception, impair your judgement and even trigger anxiety or paranoia,' I explained, my gaze sweeping across the attentive faces of my audience. 'Regular use can also interfere with brain development, especially in adolescents, leading to long-term cognitive deficits and memory problems.'[2]

'Ganja,' 'pot,' 'weed,' 'cannabis'—call it whatever you like, the harm it does remains the same. Many people believe marijuana is healthier than smoking cigarettes, but research shows that both can have significant negative impacts[3] on health (to understand the impact of smoking, check page 83).

A collective murmur of concern rippled through the room, prompting me to press on with my impromptu lecture on the perils of substance abuse.

'Furthermore, smoking marijuana can irritate your lungs and respiratory system, increasing your risk of bronchitis and other respiratory infections,'[4] I continued, my voice tinged with urgency. 'And let's not forget the legal ramifications. Possession and use of marijuana are illegal[5] in our country, with serious legal consequences for those caught in possession.'

As my words sank in, I could sense a palpable shift in the atmosphere, the gravity of my message resonating with each member of the group. Gone were the frivolous plans and idle chatter, replaced by a newfound awareness of the potential dangers lurking behind the allure of recreational drugs.

Soon someone said, 'Never have I ever . . . danced in the rain!'

This was followed by squeals and shrieks as all of them ran to the balcony to dance in the rain.

Why Should Earbuds Come with a 'Handle with Care' Warning?

Earbuds: those tiny, fluffy sticks that most of us keep in our bathrooms, thinking they're harmless and, indeed, helpful for cleaning our ears.

These little tools are used by a whopping 79.6 per cent of people, even though they come with a concerning 2.4 per cent injury rate[1] despite their seemingly innocent appearance.

But here's the twist—these earbuds might be doing more harm than good! Surprised? Well, there are more revelations ahead.

First off, let's give earwax some credit. It's not just some gross gunk; it actually has a purpose. Earwax, or cerumen if you want to get fancy, is like the body's own bouncer. And it actually has a job to do!

1. **Protection:** It traps dust, dirt and other particles, stopping them from getting to your eardrum.[2]
2. **Lubrication:** It keeps the skin in your ear canal nice and moist, preventing dryness and itching.[3]

3. **Antibacterial properties:** Earwax is like a tiny germ-fighting superhero, helping to prevent infections.[4]

Normally, earwax makes its way out of the ear on its own. Most people don't need to clean their ears at all.

Here's where things get tricky. When you use an earbud, you often push the earwax deeper into the ear canal rather than getting it out. And that's where the problems start:

1. **Impacted earwax:** Shoving earwax deeper can cause it to build up and get stuck. This can make your ear feel full, lead to hearing loss and sometimes requires a trip to the doctor to fix.
2. **Injury:** The ear canal and eardrum are delicate. Sticking an earbud in too far can cause scratches, or even worse, can perforate your eardrum. This can also cause eardrum perforation and stuck objects.[5] Ouch!
3. **Infection:** Introducing bacteria into your ear canal with an earbud can lead to nasty ear infections.[6]

Many people think earbuds are designed for cleaning ears, but in reality, they are intended for external use only, such as applying or removing makeup or cleaning around the outer ear. They should not be used to clean inside the ear canal. Most brands even have warnings about not sticking them in your ear canal, such as this one:

CAUTION: Do not enter the ear canal. Use only as directed. Entering the ear canal could cause injury. Keep out of reach of children.

But who reads those, right? Despite these warnings, many folks still use them wrong, simply because the little sticks are everywhere and old habits die hard.

So if earbuds aren't the answer, what is? Here are some better options:

1. **Let nature do its thing**: The easiest and safest option is to do nothing. Your body will take care of earwax removal naturally.
2. **Visit a pro**: If earwax buildup is an issue, see an ENT specialist. They have the right tools and the knowledge to clean your ears safely.
3. **Ear drops**: Over-the-counter ear drops can help soften earwax, making it easier for your body to expel it.

So the next time you reach for an earbud, remember, it's not a tiny magic wand for ear hygiene. Think twice and give your ears a break from your DIY medical skills. Your ears will thank you for the gentle care they deserve!

Milk vs Dark

A Sweet Showdown of Chocolate Misconceptions

I love family get-togethers. Love, laughter and endless banter are all they stand for. My cousin Payal was coming to India after three years and we had planned a special gathering for her.

Last Sunday was the day of the family gathering and the house was bustling with activity. Laughter, chatter and the aroma of homemade delicacies filled the air, enticing everyone's taste buds.

'Manan beta, aren't you having any kheer?' my Mami asked, noticing my empty dessert plate.

I smiled politely and declined, 'No thank you, Mami. I'm trying to cut back on sugar.'

'Arre, as a child you used to love the kheer I make. Please have just one bowl.' She shook her head and tried to make me eat one bowl of kheer. I kept on refusing.

After a little bit of cajoling, she quit asking me and moved on to other interested participants who cared for a refill of the kheer.

Soon after lunch, we all were sitting in the lounge. On the centre table was a huge bowl full of chocolates that

Payal had brought. As the conversations flowed, everyone kept grabbing one chocolate after another.

I looked carefully in the bowl and picked a dark chocolate for myself. I had just taken one bite when my Mami saw this and got angry: 'Manan, this is so wrong. When I insisted you have kheer, you refused, saying you are cutting down on sugar. And now, you are having chocolate? I am hurt!'

'But Mami . . . this is dark chocolate . . .' I tried to defend myself.

Before I could elaborate, my cousin Riya interjected, her tone sceptical, 'Isn't dark chocolate just as unhealthy as milk chocolate?'

'No! On the contrary, dark chocolate is quite different from milk chocolate,' I told them.

Dark chocolate has enormous health benefits. It contains several health-promoting factors, bio-active components and vitamins and minerals that positively modulate the immune system of human beings.[1]

It safeguards against cardiovascular disease certain types of cancers and other brain-related disorders like Alzheimer's disease, Parkinson's disease, etc.[2]

Dark chocolate is considered a functional food due to its anti-diabetic, anti-inflammatory and anti-microbial properties. It also has a well-established role in weight management and the alteration of a lipid profile to a healthy direction. [3]

Mohit, who had been silently observing the conversation, chimed in, 'I've heard that dark chocolate can improve brain function too. Is that true?'

I nodded, impressed by his knowledge. 'Yes, absolutely! Dark chocolate contains caffeine and theobromine, which can enhance cognitive function[4] and boost the mood.[5] Plus, it stimulates the release of endorphins, also known as "feel-good" hormones, which can help alleviate stress and improve overall well-being.[6] Just make sure you don't consume more than 100gm[7] of dark chocolate per week.'

As I spoke, I noticed the scepticism fading from Riya's face, replaced by genuine curiosity. 'Wow, I had no idea dark chocolate had so many health benefits. But what about the sugar content?'

I smiled, anticipating her question. 'While dark chocolate does contain some sugar, it's typically less than milk chocolate. The higher cocoa content means it has a richer flavour, so you don't need to consume as much to satisfy your sweet cravings. Always insist on having dark chocolate with 80 per cent cocoa[8] only!'

Mami nodded thoughtfully and said, 'Time to learn how to make dark chocolate cookies for Manan now!'

As everyone laughed, I understood that day that her love language was food.

Bubble Trouble

The Truth About the Sulphate-Free Shampoo Hype

Last weekend, as I strolled down the supermarket, my eyes scanned the colourful array of products neatly stacked on the shelves. Suddenly, I spotted my neighbours, Mr and Mrs Khanna, in a nearby row. Intrigued, I made my way over to greet them.

'Hello!' I exclaimed, smiling warmly as Mr Khanna extended his hand for a shake. They were always inseparable, but today they seemed to be arguing about something.

Mr Khanna turned to his wife and said, 'Let's ask him. He's a doctor; he'll know better.' Then he turned to me and said, 'Dr Manan, we're debating which shampoo to buy. My wife wants to get a sulphate-free shampoo after seeing all those ads on TV, but I'm dead against it. I've read some terrible things about it.'

I looked at Mrs Khanna.

'Yes, I've heard that sulphate-free shampoos are better for your hair. They're supposed to be gentler and less harsh,' Mrs Khanna explained, looking thoughtful.

'Well, actually . . .' I hesitated for a bit before blurting out, 'sulphate-free shampoos have their own pros and cons.'

Mrs Khanna looked surprised.

Let's first look at why sulphates are important in shampoo. Sulphates assist shampoo in removing oil and dirt from the hair. However, the hair needs to maintain some of its natural moisture and oils to remain healthy. Otherwise, it can cause dryness of the scalp and irritation.[1] This removal of excessive moisture results in dry and unhealthy hair.[2]

'Removing sulphate from shampoos would mean less lather. It would also cause less damage to the scalp and hair. Sulphate-free shampoos can keep the hair clean and nourished. They also help in achieving stronger, softer and shinier locks. Sulphate-free shampoos also help maintain the colour of dyed hair,'[3] I explained and added, 'However, they are known to leave the hair greasy.'[4]

Many sulphate-free shampoos are made with milder, gentler ingredients, but not all of them are. Some of them use mild cleansers[5] like decyl glucoside or coco glucoside. While they're gentle on delicate scalps and hair, they often can't remove the product build-up that many people have, which not only leaves the hair greasy, but can also be harmful in the long run.

I looked at Mr Khanna, who had an 'I-said-so' look on his face.

'But seeing those ads about breakage and hair fall, I thought this would prevent me from going bald,' Mrs Khanna remarked with a sombre expression.

I was concerned now. 'Mrs Khanna, haircare is not one-size-fits-all. Shampoos are not medicated magic that deliver on their promises as shown in the ads. If the hair fall is severe, it's advisable to consult a dermatologist or a trichologist.[6] They can assess your scalp and hair condition and recommend products that are medically approved and suited to your specific needs.'

Mrs Khanna was lost in thought for a few moments.

'Why don't we stick to our good old shampoo until we stumble upon a better alternative and maybe a decent dermatologist?' Mr Khanna suggested, his grin widening mischievously as he held up a shampoo bottle.

Mrs Khanna couldn't help but give in. 'Alright, alright, you win. Looks like we're sticking to our usual shampoo after all.'

Cracking the Egg Joke

Sunny Side Up on Cholesterol Fables

A pproaching the topic of egg consumption is as fragile as handling their shells. Proceed with caution.

No matter your age, shape or hustle, you'll always hear the same old tune: 'Stay away from those egg yolks, they're trouble!' But are egg yolks really harmful?

Let me be your Watson today and investigate the truth behind this intricate web of cautionary tales.

Despite the egg yolk's cholesterol reputation, it seems the cholesterol inside eggs isn't throwing any health tantrums.[1] And as it turns out, egg yolks are innocent! No need to blame them for cholesterol[2] anymore.

So, should you have it? Absolutely!

Incorporating egg yolks into your daily diet is a health-positive decision, supported by abundant evidence. It's more than elementary!

How many?

Well, apparently, the egg yolk rulebook seems to be missing a few pages. They can't decide whether to crack down on yolks or let them run free like sunny-side-up rebels!

Time to crack an egg and look at the pros closely. Egg yolk boasts a hefty load of lipids, which make up about 33 per cent of its entirety. While triglycerides take the lead among these lipids, egg yolk stands out as the richest source of phospholipids and dietary cholesterol.[3]

More than 95 per cent of the cholesterol found in egg yolk is classified as free cholesterol, serving a crucial function in upholding the structure of lipoproteins.[4] Despite its bad rap, cholesterol is actually the unsung hero of the body. It's the glue that holds our cell membranes together and the mastermind behind our hormone production, bile acid synthesis and vitamin D creation.

Remember the feeling of fullness it induces? The satiety effect of egg protein from the yolk is notably higher compared to other protein sources.[5]

Choline is an important nutrient necessary for foetal and neonatal brain development. For pregnant and lactating mothers, egg yolks can be a great source of this nutrient.[6]

The phosvitin found in egg yolk serves as a natural bioactive compound inhibiting hyperpigmentation in human skin.[7]

A protein-rich diet with egg yolks is like a match made in heaven. They'll keep you feeling full and fuelled as you cruise through the day. Packed with some amazing health benefits, they are also a great way to cut down on fat.

So friends, leave behind your worries and have egg yolks for breakfast and curries!

From Tennis Courts to Cubicles

The Truth About Tennis Elbow

As I settled into my clinic, I was greeted by the familiar face of an old client, Mrs Rao, a forty-five-year-old homemaker. One look at her face and I knew she was in discomfort. 'What brings you here today, Mrs Rao?' I asked, motioning for her to take a seat.

Mrs Rao replied, 'Doc, I've been having this terrible pain in my elbow for the past few days. It's really bothering me, and I haven't done anything to injure it. I am unable to lift even a bottle of water.'

Moving on to the elbow, I touched it softly and Mrs Rao grimaced in pain. I noticed that her expression changed as I applied pressure to the specific tendon that connects the muscles to the bone on the outside of the elbow.

I put my thumb at that exact tendon origin without applying pressure and asked Mrs Rao, 'Is the pain located on the outside of your elbow? Does it worsen when you grip or lift objects?'

Mrs Rao nodded vigorously. 'Yes, that is the place.'

With a gentle smile, I explained, 'Well, Mrs Rao, it sounds like you might be experiencing a condition called tennis elbow.'

'Tennis elbow?' Mrs Rao exclaimed in surprise. 'But I don't even play tennis. I have never even held a tennis racquet in my life, Doctor!'

Chuckling, I reassured her, 'You don't have to be a tennis player to get tennis elbow. It's a common condition that can affect anyone, regardless of whether or not they play sports.'[1]

Mrs Rao looked intrigued, so I continued, 'Tennis elbow, or lateral epicondylitis is caused by overuse of the forearm muscles and tendons.[2] It can happen to people who perform repetitive motions with their arms and hands, such as typing, painting, gardening, or lifting weights.[3] Or even to homemakers, because many household chores[4] include repetitive movements that can cause tennis elbow.'

Tennis elbow can develop gradually over time, so it's not uncommon for people to experience it without realizing the cause.

Mrs Rao looked a bit relieved but still concerned. 'Is it serious, Doc? Will it affect my work and daily activities?'

'Not to worry, Mrs Rao,' I reassured her. 'Tennis elbow is usually a self-limiting condition, meaning it tends to improve on its own with time and proper care.'[5]

I went on to explain, 'The first step is to rest the affected arm and avoid activities that aggravate the pain.[6] You can also apply ice packs to reduce inflammation. I will also give you some painkillers to reduce your discomfort.'[7]

When working long hours at a desk, it's crucial to have an ergonomic chair and desk that provide adequate support for your arms, back and neck to prevent such complaints.

Mrs Rao listened attentively, nodding along as I spoke. 'Additionally,' I continued, 'physiotherapy[8] can help strengthen the forearm muscles and improve flexibility.'

As I wrote a prescription for her, Mrs Rao heaved a sigh of relief and said, 'I now understand how important it is to see a doctor and not ignore any health issues for long. The Internet can scare you after a point!'

Scoops of Lies

The Cold Conspiracy of Ice Cream

One weekend, my father's friend paid him a visit along with his eight-year-old grandchild, Rahul. Initially excited about the new environment, the child soon grew bored and sat gloomily in a corner. It was sweltering and even indoors felt cramped. Wanting to cheer him up, I offered him ice cream.

'I have a cold. Mamma said I shouldn't eat ice cream,' Rahul replied, on the verge of tears.

'Eating ice cream won't make your cold worse,' I assured him. Suddenly, the room fell silent, and everyone's attention turned to me.

I glanced at their inquisitive expressions and felt a wave of apprehension wash over me. The excitement in the room was palpable. Shifting from global economics and national politics, my audience's attention was now laser-focused on the mysteries of ice cream.

I ushered the child to the centre of the couch and took a seat beside him, fully committed to unravelling the enigma of ice cream.

Cold is basically a viral infection that impacts the upper respiratory tract.[1] It is the most common viral infection that almost everybody gets. Roughly 25 per cent of all types of colds remain unexplained by proven causes.[2]

Suddenly the kid sneezed, '*Acchhoo* . . .'

I offered him a tissue paper to clean his nose and said, 'When we catch a cold, our body naturally produces a slippery discharge known as mucus, leading to congestion. Ice cream contains milk, and some folks think milk triggers mucus production. That's a misconception.'[3]

'But Dr Manan,' Rahul pointed to his throat and said, '*Kuch Kuch Hota Hai* (a popular Bollywood movie whose name translates to "Something is happening")!'

I replied with utmost seriousness, struggling to contain my laughter, '*Tum nahi samjhoge*, Rahul. *Kuch nahi hota hai!*'

'Manan, how on earth could that be? We've been hearing this since we were kids and I know for a fact that the mucus becomes thicker when you eat ice cream,' complained Raman Uncle, my dad's buddy, with a hint of irritation.

'That is because ice cream or any dairy product makes the phlegm thicker. There is no other reason behind it.'[4]

Did You Know?

Ice cream is often recommended for children immediately after tonsil removal surgery to help **alleviate their pain.**[5]

Ice cream contains milk and milk solids, offering vital nutrients such as vitamin D, vitamin A, calcium, phosphorus and riboflavin.[6] For e.g., dark chocolate ice cream is rich in antioxidants and flavonoids, which have been shown to reduce LDL cholesterol levels and enhance heart health.[7] Ice cream provides important and essential elements.[8]

However, one must not forget the sugar content and the calories in an ice cream.

'All this chatter about ice cream is really tempting me to indulge in one right now. Anyone else feeling the same cravings?' Raman Uncle queried, a mischievous grin spreading across his face.

A resounding 'yes' reverberated throughout the room.

I took Rahul piggyback as we walked towards the kitchen to get ice cream for everyone and sang, 'I scream, you scream, we all scream for ice cream' together.

Thirty-Day Weight Loss

Miracle or Mischief?

My childhood friend Raj was getting married to Anita, his long-term girlfriend. They had been college sweethearts. Staying in the same building as Raj meant witnessing their love story in many ways.

From orchestrating the proposal to breaking the news to his parents, and now with the impending wedding on the horizon, I've been there every step of the way. For the past few weeks, our weekends have been filled with shopping excursions followed by leisurely relaxation sessions at either of our homes.

One evening, as we lounged on his couch, munching on snacks and reminiscing about old times, he dropped a bombshell.

'So, Manan, you won't believe what Anita's up to now,' Raj said, his eyes wide.

'What's she done now?' I asked, raising an eyebrow.

'She's only gone and signed up for a thirty-day weight loss programme!' Raj exclaimed, his tone a mix of disbelief and admiration.

I chuckled, shaking my head in mock disbelief. 'Oh, the classic pre-wedding fitness frenzy. I've seen it all before.'

'Yeah, but the thing is, she wants me to do it too,' Raj confessed, his expression shifting from amusement to uncertainty.

I raised an eyebrow, giving him a pointed look. 'And are you seriously considering it?'

Raj shrugged, looking torn. 'I mean, she's really into it, and I guess it wouldn't hurt to shed a few pounds before the big day, right?'

I leaned back, contemplating his dilemma. 'Listen, Raj, I get that you want to look your best for the wedding, but let me tell you something. Those thirty-day workout challenges? They might give you some quick results, but they're not sustainable in the long run.'[1]

Trendy diets are not the answer to achieving weight loss.[2]

Raj furrowed his brow, clearly intrigued by my words. 'What do you mean?'

'All I am saying is fitness isn't a thirty-day challenge, my friend. It's a lifelong journey. Sure, you might see some changes in a month, but real longevity benefits[3] come from thinking long-term.'

Achieving lasting weight loss requires individuals to perceive it as a life-long commitment.[4]

Raj nodded thoughtfully, soaking in my words. 'So you're saying I shouldn't bother with the thirty-day programme?'

I shook my head, a playful grin spreading across my face. 'I'm saying you should focus on building healthy habits[5] that you can sustain for the rest of your life. That means regular exercise, balanced nutrition and plenty of rest.'[6]

After a brief pause, I added, 'Losing weight in 30 days? More like a fairy tale! But why not see it as the first step in your journey to forming a workout habit? Use this time to explore which exercises you actually enjoy and what suits your body best. Stick with it beyond the 30 days, and you might just find yourself on the road to better health!'

Raj sighed, rubbing his temples in frustration. 'But it's so tempting to go for the quick fix, you know? Especially when the wedding is just around the corner.'

I reached out, placing a reassuring hand on his shoulder. 'I know it's tempting, Raj, but trust me, it's not worth sacrificing your long-term health for short-term gains.[7] Instead of focusing on losing weight for the wedding, why not focus on becoming the healthiest version of yourself?'

Raj nodded slowly, a determined glint entering his eyes. 'You're right, Manan. I want to be healthy and happy, not just for the wedding, but for the rest of my life.'

'Yes, bro! And this advice isn't just for you; it's for your future better half too. After all, you both need to be in tune!' I suggested.

Raj confessed, 'You know, Manan, we figured this 30-day programme would give us some extra quality time together before the wedding chaos kicks in. You know how crazy it gets as the big day approaches. But now, with all this newfound wisdom, I am confused about how to break this news to her!'

'Why don't we kick off rehearsals for your sangeet? It's not just great cardio, but also a ton of fun. Plus, I must fulfil my childhood dream of dancing to *Mere Yaar Ki Shaadi Hai* . . . at your wedding,' I instantly said.

Raj promptly got up from the couch and took his phone from the table.

'What? Where?' I asked.

'Got to make calls. Anita. Then a choreographer. We have just a month left, you see!' Raj smiled and winked.

Finally, the wedding madness had begun!

X-Rated Reality

Debunking the Illusion of Harmless Porn

It was a typical afternoon and I was catching up with my friend Shyam over coffee at our favourite cafe. We were engrossed in conversation when suddenly Shyam's phone rang, startling him.

He glanced at the caller ID and sighed before reluctantly answering the call. 'Hey, Mom,' he greeted, his tone wary.

I couldn't help but overhear bits and pieces of the conversation as Shyam's expression shifted from annoyance to concern. It seemed that his younger brother was in a sticky situation—caught red-handed watching porn.

I exchanged a sympathetic glance with Shyam as he listened to his mother's tirade on the other end of the line. She was clearly not happy about the situation and wanted Shyam to intervene and set his brother straight.

But Shyam wasn't having it. 'Mom, come on, it's not a big deal,' he protested, his frustration evident in his voice. 'Every guy watches porn at some point. It's natural curiosity.'

I watched as Shyam's face flushed with anger at his mother's response. 'Fine, whatever,' he snapped, ending the call abruptly.

I could tell Shyam was agitated, so I decided to weigh in on the matter. 'Hey, Shyam, I know you're upset, but maybe there's more to this than meets the eye,' I ventured cautiously.

Shyam looked at me, clearly intrigued. 'What do you mean?' he asked, his curiosity piqued.

'Well, you know, there are actually several reasons why watching porn can be harmful,' I explained, leaning in earnestly. 'For starters, it can create unrealistic expectations[1] about sex and relationships, which can lead to dissatisfaction and disappointment in real-life experiences.'

The majority of studies indicate that porn addiction is classified as a form of substance abuse.[2] The effects of pornography are diverse and intricate. Actors are frequently seen as victims of abuse and exploitation, while audience members are often criticized for becoming desensitized to sexual violence. Additionally, some argue that pornography perpetuates harmful racial and gender stereotypes.[3]

Shyam nodded thoughtfully, absorbing my words. 'Yeah, I can see how that could be a problem,' he admitted. 'But is that it?'

I shook my head. 'Not at all,' I replied. 'Pornography often depicts sex in a way that's disconnected from emotions and intimacy, focusing solely on physical pleasure. This can distort one's understanding of healthy sexuality and contribute to issues like objectification and misogyny.'

Moreover, many studies have also discussed the psychological impacts of pornography, including feelings of sadness,[4] depression, low self-esteem and loss of appetite.[5]

Shyam's eyes widened in realization. 'Wow, I never thought about it like that,' he said, his voice tinged with surprise.

'And don't forget about addiction. That can be a big problem too.'

Pornography can be highly addictive and individuals with pornography addiction often experience higher rates of general anxiety, psychological distress and weakened emotional connections[6] with family members.

Shyam looked solemn as he processed this information. 'I had no idea,' he admitted quietly. 'I guess I need to have a serious talk with my brother about this and make sure he understands the risks.'

I patted Shyam on the back in solidarity. 'Yes, bro! That's the right approach,' I reassured him with a supportive smile. 'We all have been through that phase in life. But with a friendly approach, you can help him make informed choices and navigate this complex aspect of growing up.'

Conclusion

As I conclude this book, I can't help but feel a sense of satisfaction and hope.

Together, we've embarked on a journey filled with laughter, learning and a few surprises along the way. We've explored the ins and outs of health and wellness, debunked countless myths and shared more than a few laughs.

But amidst the jokes and anecdotes lies something deeper: hope.

I hope that:

- No illness is insurmountable.
- No matter your age, it's never too late to start prioritizing your health.
- No pain is too great to heal from.
- No matter what health challenges you may face, there's always a path forward.
- With the right knowledge and guidance, you can overcome any obstacle that comes your way.

I hope this book:

- Serves as a reminder that you are capable of achieving the health and wellness you desire.

- Encourages you to take that first step towards a healthier, fitter version of yourself.
- Empowers you to question everything you read or hear, to seek science and logic in all that is shared with you.

In today's world, where knowledge is just a click away, so is misinformation. From WhatsApp forwards touting miraculous quick fixes to Instagram's self-proclaimed health gurus promising instant cures, the abundance of misinformation can be daunting.

With an endless stream of content available at our fingertips, it's more important than ever to discern fact from fiction. In this chaotic swirl of information overload, it's crucial to rely on evidence-based knowledge as our ultimate guide.

Science, with its rigorous methods and proven facts, stands as the bedrock of reliable information. It employs systematic processes to test hypotheses, validate theories and uncover truths about the natural world. This approach ensures that the knowledge we gain is accurate and dependable. By trusting in science, we can steer clear of the falsehoods and half-truths that float around social media and online forums.

Let this book be your shield against the clutches of misinformation. It will equip you with the tools to critically evaluate the claims you encounter daily. By grounding you in the reality that only science can offer, this book will help you navigate the complexities of modern information, ensuring that you make informed decisions based on solid evidence and not on unverified claims or misleading anecdotes.

As you move forward, I hope you'll keep this book close at hand, referring to it whenever you need a bit of guidance or reassurance. Remember, you have the power to take control of your health and your life.

So here's to you, dear reader. Here's to your health and happiness. And here's to the future, filled with endless possibilities and boundless hope.

Acknowledgements

They say it takes a village to bring a book to life, and they're right. Though I'd need another book to thank everyone, these are the pillars that made this journey possible.

My parents, who never dictated my choices, or my sister's, but always encouraged us to trust our instincts and strive for the best. This book carries a piece of you in every word.

My grandparents from both sides of the family—your unwavering love and countless life lessons during my upbringing have been the foundation of my strength and perseverance.

Divya—my best friend turned wife who's been my lifelong cheerleader, believing in me even when I doubted myself and always answering my wildest ideas with a simple, unwavering, 'Just do it!'

My sister **Urvi** for her endless encouragement, brother-in-law **Deepam** for his steadfast support and my nephew **Mehaan** for his infectious energy.

Messi—the best furry co-author a writer could ask for. Your loyalty and playful spirit kept me motivated and inspired throughout this journey.

Sakshi—my strategist cum mastermind behind every move, who turned plans into actions and made sure everything fell into place.

Deepthi, Manish and the entire team at Penguin Random House India—your expertise made this journey smoother than I could have imagined. Thank you for believing in me and making this book shine.

Arnav and his brilliant crew at **In a Giffy** for their invaluable help in conceptualizing this book. Your insights and support truly made all the difference!

Namrata, the sounding board of the project—your support and perspective were key to its development.

Anushka, Om, AJ, Manya, Vineeka, Dhruv, Janhavi, Pratichi, Adi, Sid, Ruchi and Surabhi—thank you for being an integral part of my growth on social media, this book would never be happening if it wasn't for your contribution throughout my journey.

To all the members of the **Sheth and Pherwani families**, your faith in my abilities has been the wind beneath my wings, making this accomplishment possible.

As this book was heading to print, we were blessed with our greatest chapter yet—becoming parents to **Krish**! Juggling final edits with newborn snuggles, we've learned that the best stories are the ones life writes for us.

My incredible online community—it's been quite a ride, from those humble beginnings on Instagram to this moment of publishing a book. Your unwavering support and enthusiasm have been the highlight of this journey. Every interaction, every word of encouragement and every piece of advice you shared have shaped this book in ways words can't fully express. Looking back, I'm deeply grateful for the role each of you played. Thanks for sticking with me from the start and for making this journey so memorable. This book is for YOU.

To all those who aren't mentioned by name but who have been just as crucial—your support has been like the hidden threads in a tapestry, you might not always be seen, but your influence is woven into every page.

Notes

Scan QR code to go to the Notes section of the book at https://drmananvora.com/but-what-does-science-say/ notes.

Scan QR code to access the
Penguin Random House India website